ALCOHOL ABUSE

HOW TO HELP A LOVED ONE

Pippa Sales

Disa Publications

Alcohol Abuse: How To Help A Loved One
Copyright © 1994 by Pippa Sales

Published by Disa Publications
350 Ward Avenue, Suite 106
Honolulu, HI 96814

Printed in the United States of America

Library of Congress Cataloging in Publication Data

Sales, Pippa
    Alcohol abuse : how to help a loved one / Pippa Sales.
    p. cm.
    Includes bibliographical references.
    Preassigned LCCN: 94-094058.
    ISBN 1-884633-01-3

    1. Alcoholism. 2. Alcoholism--Treatment. 3. Alcoholics.
4. Alcoholics--Family relationships.   I. Title.

HV5275.S354 1994   362.292'3
                                         QBI94-439

For my family and friends
with love and thanks

They can because they think they can

Warning and Disclaimer

The author and publisher disclaim all liability in connection with the use and/or implementation of any information from this book.

The views expressed in this book are a summary of some of the popular current beliefs on alcoholism as expressed by experts in the field of alcoholism.

The author and publisher are not responsible for any action taken as a result of reading this book. This book is intended as a general guide — an introduction to the disease of alcoholism and what can be done about it. This book is not a substitute for medical advice from a licensed physician or other professional trained in alcoholism.

A listing in the resource section does not represent an endorsement from the author or publisher. Neither do the author and publisher endorse any of the resource listings. The addresses and telephone numbers were current at the time of writing. The author and publisher regret any inconvenience due to any subsequent changes.

Contents

Foreword

When we ponder the various epidemics, diseases and plagues that have swept human populations throughout history, an eerie chill and a feeling of powerlessness overcome us. It is not surprising, therefore, that we take great pride and comfort in the accomplishment of modern scientific research and the hope it holds in finding cures and preventative measures for the diseases and the "curses" that visit mankind from time to time.

We always look and listen for news of breakthroughs in the search for cures to cancer, heart disease and AIDS. And we examine, treat and innoculate our bodies in an effort to avoid such illnesses. Yet, at this very moment, one out of ten Americans is suffering from a widely ignored, progressive and potentially fatal disease. Very few of those afflicted are aware of their disease. Some of those afflicted will die and with their last breath deny the existence of this disease. This disease is alcoholism.

Alcoholism is not just a disease of the poor; it is not related to lack of proper sanitation or nutrition, although those living in poverty are also affected. Some studies suggest that the higher a person's education, the greater a person's income, the greater the incidence of the disease.

Surveys done by several Bar Associations indicate that from 15 to 20 percent of lawyers are or will become alcoholics. That fact has always puzzled me. In my work counseling attorneys and judges I have learned of their interest in maintaining good health. They show concern about their weight, their cholesterol levels and blood pressure. They have access to the finest medical care available. So how is it that they do not take action against this life-destroying disease?

I believe that there are two main reasons. The first is lack of education of the symptoms, the progression, the nature of the disease itself and the treatment available. The second reason is inherent in the nature of the illness. Alcoholism is not only a devastating disease. Alcoholism carries with its destructiveness a very effective mechanism which hides the disease from the awareness of the victim. This defense is called denial.

Denial makes it almost impossible for the alcoholic to realize the mental, physical, emotional and spiritual debilitation he or she may be enduring. The alcoholic is usually the last person in the world to acknowledge the extent of his or her addiction.

If we, as a caring society, wish to arrest this epidemic we must educate not only the alcoholics but more importantly those around the alcoholics who can lead them out of the darkness of denial.

It is exactly for this purpose that Pippa Sales has written *Alcohol Abuse: How To Help A Loved One*. Pippa has addressed most of the significant issues pertaining to alcoholism and recovery in a clear and concise manner. Her book will be a great help to many people in the community who are suffering from alcoholism — or who have friends or relatives suffering. The brief and clear language in this book will make sense to all affected by alcoholism, even those who are so emotionally entangled with the disease that they thought help was beyond hope.

Pippa's efforts should be of great benefit to society.

Peter A. Donahoe, J.D., Director
Attorneys and Judges Assistance Program
Supreme Court, State of Hawaii

1

The Cost Of Alcoholism To The Nation

"Alcohol can kill."

Alcoholism is not just a disease. Alcoholism is the number one health problem in the United States. Alcoholism is the number two killer in the United States after cancer. There are over 18 million alcoholics in the United States. Alcohol probably kills more people each year than all illegal drugs combined. Alcohol is the most commonly abused drug in our society. The economic cost to society of alcohol dependency and alcoholism is estimated to be close to $100 billion.

In short, people die from alcoholism and the cost to the nation is quite staggering.

For each person that has the disease of alcoholism, at least four other people are directly affected by that person's alcoholism. That is a lot of people suffering in this country. The tragedy is that few people do anything about their own or another person's alcoholism. Or, they wait until the disease is so far advanced that the person suffering from alcoholism is severely physically and mentally harmed.

You CAN do something about alcoholism. The sooner you help an alcoholic to treatment the greater the chance of recovery. Alcoholism is the most untreated treatable disease in the United States. Often the people closest to the alcoholic find it hardest to see and admit that someone they care about is an alcoholic. These people, however, are the very ones who can help to break the vicious cycle of the disease and are in the position to intervene. How long do you want to watch the self destruction of a loved one?

In spite of all the trouble that drinking may have caused, few people want to admit that someone they love is an alcoholic. There has been a stigma attached to the word. No more. No need to feel ashamed. It is a disease like any other disease and needs to be treated. It is a disease just as heart disease, cancer or diabetes are diseases. If someone you love had one of these diseases, you would get treatment for that person, wouldn't you?

Guide your loved one to help for his or her alcoholism. The deceptive nature of the disease makes it hard for alcoholics to recognize their problem or do anything about it. The disease allows the alcoholic to live in a state of denial. If you accept this denial, the alcoholic could die. The alcoholic needs a helping hand to get to treatment and onto the road of recovery.

This book is for those of you who have a dependency on alcohol and for those of you who love someone who is dependent on alcohol. The goal of this book is to offer you:

- a better understanding of alcoholism and why alcoholics have difficulty in seeking the help they desperately need;

- how it affects both alcoholics and those closest to them;

- how you can do something to guide the alcoholic to treatment by Intervention;

- and, most importantly, where you can find help in the area where you live.

If each one of us helped guide one alcoholic to treatment, we would not only be helping that one person but the whole nation. With fewer alcoholics drinking, we would live in a much safer country. We would have fewer car accidents, less crime, less spouse and child abuse, less property destruction, less fire destruction, and fewer people in jails.

We can measure the financial cost to society of alcoholism, but we cannot measure the pain, suffering and family disruptions that it causes. Why suffer any more? Get help — for you and the alcoholic.

There is plenty of in-depth literature on alcoholism. Get it and read it if you want to know more. This book is a start, a simple guide to get you to DO something to help yourself or a loved one; to do something before a disaster strikes. You do not want anyone you know to become a statistic. There is so much help available that there is no reason why you cannot get help NOW!

Bacchus has drowned more men than Neptune.

— Guiseppe Garibaldi

2

The Disease of Alcoholism

"Nobody wants to become an alcoholic."

What is alcoholism?

Alcoholism is a powerful, life-threatening disease.

A person with alcoholism is physically dependent on alcohol. The nature of the disease affects the body and brain in such a way that the person has no control over his or her drinking. In fact, the drinking controls the alcoholic.

Alcoholism is a chronic, progressive and primary disease.

By chronic it is meant that the disease is long lasting and there is no known cure for it. Alcoholism can be controlled by not drinking and is regarded as the most untreated treatable disease in the United States.

By progressive it is meant that the disease will only worsen over time. Alcoholism tends to progress through set stages — early, middle and late — with some alcoholics showing more extreme symptoms than others.

By primary it is meant that alcoholism is a disease itself and not caused by a social, emotional, or physical problem.

Alcoholism is a serious disease that needs to be treated. Understanding that alcoholism is a disease helps us to get help for the alcoholic and to treat him or her as we would a cancer or heart disease sufferer.

What is an alcoholic?

An alcoholic is a person who suffers from the disease of alcoholism.

Alcoholics are people who have become dependent on alcohol because their bodies are incapable of processing alcohol normally. Something has gone very wrong inside their bodies and the only way the disease can be halted is by not drinking.

Who becomes an alcoholic?

The disease of alcoholism can affect anyone — it does not care how old you are, what sex you are, what color you are, what religion you belong to, or how much money you have. Most alcoholics are not the "Skid Row" stereotype but regular people with jobs, families and the usual responsibilities that go with life.

If a person doesn't drink they can't become an alcoholic. You have to drink to become an alcoholic.

What are the stages of alcoholism?

1. Early or adaptive stage: The alcoholic may appear only as a heavy drinker. Drinking may be daily or less frequent and may be heavy only occasionally.

The cells in the alcoholic's body are adapting to alcohol and allowing alcohol into the body in increasing amounts.

2. Middle or dependent stage: The cells in the alcoholic's body become dependent on alcohol. There are many alterations in the normal functioning of cells of the body and the disease can no longer remain hidden. The alcoholic is now dependent on alcohol.

3. Late or deteriorative stage: Alcohol seriously affects the alcoholic's mental, emotional and physical health. There is damage to vital organs in the body and the alcoholic has a lowered resistance to infection and other diseases. At this stage the alcoholic cannot even understand that alcohol is destroying him or her.

4. Final stage: Death.

What causes alcoholism?

Current evidence points to alcoholism being a result of hereditary and environmental factors. Research is not conclusive and is ongoing.

Why do alcoholics take up drinking?

Alcoholics start drinking for the same reasons that other people do.

Alcohol can make people feel euphoric, stimulated, relaxed, or slightly intoxicated and is used with meals, in celebratory situations, in religious ceremonies or to enhance a social occasion.

The difference between alcoholics and other drinkers is that the alcoholic will continue to drink even after the desired physical effects have been felt.

Why do alcoholics continue drinking?

They cannot help it. The nature of the disease prevents alcoholics from realizing that they are dependent on alcohol. The alcohol alters alcoholics' thinking and reasoning and "tricks" alcoholics into believing they can handle their drinking. Once the alcohol has chemically and electrically disturbed alcoholics' brains, they do not see their behavior the way others do. They do not see or accept what is happening to them.

It is important to remember that a loved one is already an alcoholic by the time he or she begins to act like an alcoholic. By the time it is evident that a loved one may be an alcoholic, the nature of the disease prevents him or her from having control over drinking. The drinking now controls your loved one. Therefore, he or she continues to drink.

Do all alcoholics drink a lot?

No. You do not have to drink a lot or over an extended period of time to develop alcoholism. The effect alcohol has on a person is a very individual reaction. Alcoholics are characterized by how they drink — for example, in an uncontrolled way — not by how much or how often.

Is anyone who has a problem with drinking or drinks a lot an alcoholic?

No. There are problem drinkers and heavy drinkers who may or may not be alcoholics. The alcoholic has a greater emotional response to alcohol, often attaching unreasonable significance to it, than the non-alcoholic problem or heavy drinker.

Both the problem drinker and heavy drinker do need help, however, in controlling their drinking to alleviate the psychological, physical and social problems caused by drinking too much.

3

Telltale Signs of Alcoholism

"There is no 'alcoholic personality'."

How do I know if I or a loved one is dependent on alcohol?

There are many telltale signs. In the lists of signs below you may find one or many that you or a loved one can relate to.

The signs listed are for all stages of alcoholism. The chances that all signs apply to you or a loved one is very unlikely.

Look hard for the one or ones that DO apply. If only one applies there can still be a problem. Don't be fooled by the fact that each alcoholic has different telltale signs. The one thing each has in common is a loss of control over drinking and a consequent deterioration in his or her life.

Recognizing the signs is the first step to realizing there is a problem and to stopping it. Remember that it is not only alcoholics that need help but problem drinkers too.

Early warning signs are:

- an increase in the FREQUENCY of drinking
- an increase in AMOUNT of alcohol consumed
- an increasing need to FEEL THE EFFECT of alcohol (to get intoxicated)

Telltale signs in the early, middle and late stages:

- finding an excuse to drink
- finding non-drinking events boring
- drinking to build confidence with other people
- getting intoxicated when you or a loved one planned not to
- drinking to relieve tension or to escape problems
- having trouble stopping after the first drink
- sneaking drinks
- gulping drinks (drinking very fast and often without mixers)
- drinking more and more to achieve the same effect
- having guilt feelings about one's drinking
- having feelings of remorse after drinking too much
- being on the defensive about one's drinking
- trying to control drinking by changing types of alcohol
- hiding alcohol
- making promises to quit and then breaking them
- lying about one's drinking
- drinking in the morning to get rid of a hangover
- drinking at work
- drinking and driving
- skipping meals when drinking

- having blackouts (that is, not remembering the next day what was said or done the night before even though you or a loved one didn't pass out)
- binge drinking
- having accidents at work or at home with damage to oneself or one's possessions
- neglecting family responsibilities
- missing days at work because of drinking
- being late for work because of drinking
- leaving work early to go drinking
- losing a job or nearly losing a job because of drinking
- showing a personality change when drinking
- missing planned family or social activities due to drinking
- a woman drinking during pregnancy
- being concerned about your or a loved one's drinking

D*id you find the above list a little overwhelming? Then take this short self-test:*

Check your answers to the following questions:

		YES	NO
1.	Do you or a loved one lose time from work or miss appointments due to drinking?	___	___
2.	Do you or a loved one sometimes binge on alcohol?	___	___
3.	Do you or a loved one sometimes feel guilty about drinking.	___	___
4.	Do you or a loved one need more and more alcohol to get intoxicated?	___	___

		YES	*NO*
5.	Do you or a loved one often regret things said or done when intoxicated?	___	___
6.	Do you or a loved one suffer loss of memory (blackouts) while or after drinking?	___	___
7.	Do you or a loved one often fail to keep promises made to control or cut down on drinking?	___	___
8.	Do you or a loved one find that drinking is harming or worrying the family?	___	___
9.	Do you or a loved one eat very little or irregularly when drinking?	___	___
10.	Do you or a loved one drink in the morning or "need" a drink to get over a hangover?	___	___

A "yes" answer to one or more of the above questions indicates that you or a loved one may be an alcoholic or on the road to becoming one. Seek professional help. A professional trained in alcoholism will help you determine if you or a loved one is an alcoholic and what you can do about it.

4

The Physical Effects of Drinking

" You can die from drinking too much. "

D rinking too much alcohol can kill you. Is your life worth that risk?

No part of your body escapes the effects of alcohol. Alcohol is a toxic drug; it is a poison to your body. When taken in large amounts over a period of time, alcohol will affect virtually every part of your body. Alcohol can have both short-term and long-term effects on the body.

W hat are the short-term effects of alcohol on the body?

Upset stomach	ever felt queasy after a "night out"?
Diarrhea	not necessarily caused by "something you ate"!

Anemia	the all too familiar "blahs" from too much partying!
Decreased fitness	remember the hangovers! Hangovers are caused by the diuretic nature of alcohol. You're all dried out!
	alcohol affects perception and coordination
	alcohol irritates the joints and weakens your muscle fiber
Skin problems	alcohol is a diuretic causing skin to dry out
	alcohol causes the blood vessels to open up making skin look blotchy and red

What are the long-term effects of drinking?

Unfortunately the list is long as the whole body is affected.

Another unfortunate fact is that little time is spent in medical school on the subject of alcoholism. Therefore, if you lie about how much you drink, do not count on your doctor to pick up that you may have an alcohol problem. Instead of getting you to stop what is causing your problem — your drinking — your doctor may treat your heart, liver or other condition while you continue to poison yourself with further drinking.

Remember that from what you have read already, you cannot treat the problems that alcohol is causing. You have to treat the primary problem — your drinking!

If you don't quit drinking too much, then, over a period of time, these are examples of parts of your body which are most commonly affected and how:

Mouth and throat	increased incidence of cancer
Stomach	ulcers and gastritis
Pancreas	increased incidence of cancer
Liver	cirrhosis of the liver is one of the top ten causes of death in the Unitd States
Blood	increased infection risks due to decreased production of white blood cells
Heart	enlargement of the heart
	abnormalities of cardiac rhythm
	congestive heart failure
	arteriosclerosis - hardening of the arteries with fatty deposits in their walls
	hypertension
Reproductive System	fetal alcohol syndrome. Maternal drinking, including even "social drinking," affect the developing fetus and can result in abnormalities and mental retardation of the newborn. The best advice for pregnant women continues to be to abstain from alcohol. Your baby is at risk!
Respiratory System	cancer of the larynx
Glands and Hormones	sugar metabolism disturbances (hypoglycemia and hyperglycemia)
Skin	dilation of blood vessels

Musculoskeletal System	osteoporosis
	various forms of arthritis
Miscellaneous effects	injuries from motor vehicle and other accidents
	malnutrition
	metabolic and immune disorders

Do you want any of the above to happen to you or a loved one? No, of course not. If the drinking is not stopped, however, then any one of the above can happen. You or your loved one could die. Not a pleasant thought, is it?

There is nothing so bad that can happen to you that a drink won't make worse.

Men are born to succeed, not to fail.
— Henry David Thoreau

5

Defenses Used By
The Alcoholic

*"They didn't serve dinner until 10 p.m.
How was I meant to stay sober?"*

W*hat is a defense?*

Basically, it is an excuse. The alcoholic, because of negative behavior caused by drinking, is vulnerable and open to criticism from relatives, friends and acquaintances. To protect himself or herself from the guilt, paranoia, and to cope with day-to-day living, the alcoholic uses a series of defense mechanisms. The number and variety of defenses increase as the disease progresses.

Why do alcoholics use defenses?

Defenses help to protect alcoholics from being hurt. Defenses help to reduce alcoholics' anxiety in the short term because, to alcoholics, defenses explain away the negative aspects of their behavior and justify the drinking.

Defenses reduce the chances that alcoholics will do anything positive about their drinking problem because defenses block the ability to see and experience reality. Alcoholics see events the way they want to. Their perception is so distorted that you can wonder if you were at the same event that an alcoholic described — even though you were!

What are some examples of defenses?

Denial

Denial is the most commonly used defense. By denying anything related to their drinking — often including the fact that they drink — alcoholics can protect themselves from pain and hurt.

Examples: "I don't care what you or anyone else thinks, I am not an alcoholic."

"Your blood tests must be wrong, I don't drink."

"I don't know whose bottles those are in my car. I told you I have given up drinking."

"What's the big deal? My drinking affects only me."

Rationalization

Alcoholics justify their drinking, how much they drink and what happens while intoxicated.

Examples: "Drinking is part of my job." (It is?)

"If I wasn't so tired and depressed the drinks wouldn't have hit me so hard."

"John was pouring strong drinks. Everyone got a little drunk."

"Everyone gets high at weddings."

"I *need* alcohol to help me sleep (to calm me down, to relax me)."

Externalization

Alcoholics often blame others — in fact, anybody — for drinking too much, for their problems and for their bad behavior. Anything to try and justify their drinking and bad behavior. The drinking, the alcoholic believes, is because of other problems in life.

Examples: "If YOU didn't nag so much, I wouldn't drink."

"My job is so frustrating."

"My boss is giving me a hard time."

"Being married to you is enough to make anyone drink!"

"With all my worries, you'd drink too."

Minimizing

Alcoholics attempt to minimize an event until it seems insignificant. Alcoholics minimize the amount they drink and the consequences of their drinking.

Examples: "I think you're overreacting to all this."

"Okay, so I had one or two drinks but it was only a small accident." (This in response to the reality of a high blood alcohol content and a totalled car!)

"No, I only screamed at her." (This in response to an obvious and witnessed beating of a spouse.)

Selective recall

Alcoholics only remember what they want to about a situation — those facts that will support their view and justify their behavior.

Example: "How could I hurt Paul's feelings? He offered to drive me home and I didn't want to offend him." (This in response to the reality of being so intoxicated that Paul had to drive his friend home.)

Euphoric recall

Alcoholics often recall only the good in a situation. Alcoholics cannot accurately remember what they said or did while intoxicated. Alcoholics remember that they were the "life and soul of the party" but not how drunk and embarrassing they were. Alcoholics remember only how good the alcohol made them feel.

Repression

Who wants to remember something that made them feel pain, shame, guilt, scared, embarrassed or angry? Sometimes it seems easier to just "forget" what really happened or what was felt rather than to deal with it.

Example: After a night out, alcoholics on waking would rather "forget" what happened the night before as it is too uncomfortable to think about.

6

Enabling: How We As A Loved One Support The Drinking

"Oh, but she doesn't drink on Wednesdays."

What *is enabling?*

Enabling is the behavior of others that protects alcoholics from the consequences of their drinking and allows them to continue drinking.

What *is an enabler?*

A person who enables is an enabler. An enabler defends the alcoholic's drinking to everyone but the alcoholic. The enabler uses the same "defenses" to the rest of the world that the alcoholic uses.

Without the support of an enabler, the alcoholic would find it difficult to continue drinking. Enabling behavior prevents both the enabler and the alcoholic from seeing the reality of the situation.

Who can be an enabler?

An enabler is anyone who helps to make excuses or covers up for the alcoholic's behavior. They can be spouses, children, parents, friends, co-workers, neighbors, bosses, employees, doctors, clergy, psychologists, social workers, teachers, nurses, police officers, lawyers and judges.

A primary enabler is a person whose cooperation is often essential to the alcoholic's continued drinking. A primary enabler is usually the one who protects both the alcoholic and other family members from the negative effects of the disease. If the primary enabler alters his or her behavior the alcoholic would probably have to face the consequences of the drinking and be forced to change because the primary enabler is no longer "fixing things."

A secondary enabler plays a less dramatic role in the perpetuation of the alcoholic's drinking. The alcoholic's employer is often a secondary enabler. The secondary enabler tends to reinforce the alcoholic's pattern of denial by not addressing the drinking or turning a "blind eye." The alcoholic is then left with the impression that his or her drinking cannot be all that bad as people would surely say something!

What is some enabling behavior?

1. Lying to family and friends about the alcoholic's drinking.

2. Making excuses for problems caused by the alcoholic's drinking.

3. Lying to the alcoholic's employer about drinking.

4. Taking on the alcoholic's responsibilities — for example, financial responsibilities.

5. Taking care of the alcoholic physically.

6. Ignoring the pain and hurt of the children.

7. Avoiding conflict with the alcoholic by "accepting" his or her excuses.

8. Not following through on the advice obtained from counselors or knowledgeable friends — those trying to help. And, not getting help.

9. Drinking with the alcoholic in the hope of keeping the drinking within limits.

10. Getting the alcoholic out of financial or legal trouble.

Why do people enable?

People enable because they think they are protecting themselves, loved ones or the alcoholic. Those enablers who are living with an alcoholic enable to hide all the problems that can come with living in an alcoholic family - for example, financial troubles, delinquency, child or spouse abuse. People enable to hide feelings of guilt, shame, inadequacy, insecurity, and resentment caused by the alcoholic's drinking.

Why must I change my enabling behavior?

If you do not change, there is little chance that the alcoholic will change. You want to get the alcoholic to treatment and to stop drinking. Your changing is a step in the right direction.

Everyone is affected by the drinking and gets trapped in the same emotional chaos as the alcoholic. You cannot do anything for the alcoholic unless you do something for yourself first. You need to take action.

It is important to realize that you have been supporting the alcoholic's drinking and that if you change then the alcoholic will be encouraged and forced to make changes too. The alcoholic has been dependent on his or her enablers to support and maintain his or her drinking. The alcoholic is more dependent on you than you are on him or her. Without you, drinking would be more difficult to maintain. It follows, therefore, that a radical change in your enabling behavior could force the alcoholic to change and seek treatment. All your enabling behavior never got the alcoholic to stop drinking in the past; don't kid yourself that enabling behavior will cause a change in the future.

For those of you that live with an alcoholic, changing the enabling behavior can be frightening because you have been around the drinking so long. A change cannot be worse than what you have lived through already. If you cannot change the alcoholic — and how you have probably tried — then change yourself. Why should you be dragged down with the alcoholic?

What can I do to change my enabling behavior?

1. Face the truth — see the reality of the situation and that the alcoholic needs outside help.

2. Learn about the disease of alcoholism.

3. Get help for yourself (professional help or Al-Anon, a support group for the family and friends of alcoholics). Treat your own problems related to the drinking. Make yourself well!

4. Identify your enabling behaviors.

5. Learn how to stop your enabling behaviors.

6. Stop focusing on the alcoholic and the problems the drinking causes.

7. Understand and practice controlling your emotions which are probably chaotic as a result of being around an alcoholic.

8. Create a healthy home environment.

9. Pursue other interests outside the home to take the focus off the alcoholic.

10. Be gentle on yourself — you are not the cause of the alcoholism.

W*hat can happen if I change my enabling behavior?*

You will be a lot happier and you may achieve what you have wanted to all along — to get the drinking to stop.

Changing your enabling behavior will give you the strength and resolve to undertake an Intervention (discussed later in chapter on Intervention) if that is what is needed to get the alcoholic into treatment. As an enabler you are only keeping the alcoholic closer to the bottle. Free of your enabling behavior, the alcoholic has more chance of getting to treatment.

Alcoholism isn't a spectator sport.
Eventually the whole family gets to play.

Rebeta-Burditt

7

15 Don'ts: If A Loved One Is An Alcoholic

Don't listen to, "If you loved me, you would call the office and say I'm sick!"

You can help a loved one take responsibility for his or her own life and drinking by following these 15 Don'ts:

1. Don't see the alcoholism as a family disgrace. It is a disease and as with other diseases, recovery is possible. Remember, no one wants to become an alcoholic.

2. Don't hide or dump bottles. The alcoholic will only find other ways of getting a drink.

3. Don't drink along with the alcoholic. It will not make the alcoholic drink less or get him or her closer to treatment. By drinking along you reinforce the habit and keep the alcoholic from seeking help for himself or herself.

4. Don't give the alcoholic responsibilities and then get angry when they are not carried out.

5. Don't punish, nag, bribe or preach to the alcoholic. It will only increase the guilt, self-hatred, self-pity and resentment and push him or her closer to the bottle. It will also force the alcoholic to lie or to make promises that cannot be kept.

6. Don't be fooled by apparent lulls in drinking. The alcoholic may be trying to get you to believe that there is no drinking problem by going "on the wagon" for a while. Things may get a little better during a non-drinking period but will only deteriorate when the drinking starts again. And it will!

7. Don't threaten the alcoholic unless you will definitely carry out the threat. If you don't carry out the threat, the alcoholic will learn that you don't mean what you say.

8. Don't make excuses for the alcoholic. Protecting the alcoholic from the consequences of drinking will only keep him or her from seeking help.

9. Don't take on the alcoholic's responsibilities. He or she needs to face the problems caused by his or her drinking, try to solve them, or face the consequences. Taking over responsibilities from alcoholics reduces their self esteem and makes them feel unworthy, unneeded, and unwanted.

10. Don't get into arguments when the alcoholic has been drinking. Neither of you can win when "crazy-making alcohol" is talking.

11. Don't demand or accept unreasonable promises from the alcoholic. Don't use the "if you loved me" routine. The alcoholic has a disease. The alcoholic has no control over drinking and the nature of the disease will only sabotage any promises made. A broken promise will only lead to more lies and distrust.

12. Don't try to protect the alcoholic from danger. Alcoholics have got to face the consequences of their drinking or else they will never get the help they need.

13. Don't get or listen to advice from friends who do not understand the disease of alcoholism. You will only become more confused and desperate. Get help from someone trained in alcoholism.

14. Don't try to handle the alcoholic and the alcoholism yourself.You cannot do it alone. Get help from a professional trained in alcoholism and get help for yourself too.

15. Don't forget to look after yourself and let the alcoholic look after himself or herself!

Although the world is full of suffering, it is also full of the overcoming of it.

Helen Keller

8

Intervention: Something More You Can Do To Help A Loved One

"You can love someone to death. If you don't intervene they could die."

You feel that you have tried everything to get your loved one to seek help for his or her drinking. You have changed your enabling behavior and your alcoholic loved one is still not motivated to seek help. You are going crazy and cannot bear to watch your loved one drink himself or herself to death. Your loved one still will not admit to having a drinking problem. You're getting desperate! You want to take some action to prevent the drinking from becoming any more serious than it already is.

There is something you can do — an Intervention.

What is an Intervention?

An Intervention is where a group of concerned people meet the alcoholic face to face with the goal of getting him or her to be evaluated by a professional trained in alcoholism and to follow the recommendation of that evaluation.

An Intervention is a loving, caring, and well rehearsed way of telling the alcoholic, in a group setting, to what extent the drinking is affecting his or her life, and your own. Your loved one is offered a set of consequences that all point to him or her being evaluated at a treatment center and entering some kind of treatment — the first step to recovery.

Intervention can be seen as creating a controlled crisis in an attempt to get the alcoholic to treatment.

Why do an Intervention?

Because nothing else has worked in getting the alcoholic to seek help for his or her drinking! And, Intervention has a very good track record.

Your loved one has a progressive illness and is physically and emotionally sick. All his or her behavior is governed by drinking. Your loved one has no control over drinking. Drinking controls him or her. Your loved one is unable to help himself or herself. The drinking problem will not go away by itself. Through an Intervention you can take action before a crisis occurs. Why wait until a crisis occurs? The sooner you can get an alcoholic to treatment, the better the chance of him or her achieving sobriety.

If you do NOT do an Intervention, your loved one could die from drinking.

Who initiates an Intervention?

Any concerned person can initiate an Intervention — a spouse, a child, a parent, a friend, an employer, an employee.

Do I have a right to intervene?

You sure do!

An Intervention is a loving and caring act. The alcoholic has no control over drinking and what it's doing to him or her. Your loved one did not choose to become an alcoholic and deserves a chance at being freed from the bottle. By intervening you are offering your loved one help; as a way to avoid death from drinking. If he or she will not seek help, then you can offer freedom through Intervention. If he or she refuses then that is his or her responsibility — you will have done everything within your power to help.

Who is involved in an Intervention?

Concerned family members and friends with the guidance of a professional — someone trained to do Intervention. Family and friends who have the greatest influence in the alcoholic's life and those who have the strongest consequences to impose are the most effective in an Intervention.

A boss or co-worker is sometimes involved because losing a job is often more threatening to the alcoholic than losing family or possessions.

What steps do I take to prepare for an Intervention?

1. Seek the assistance of a professional counselor who is trained in Intervention. Intervention is a difficult process, burdened with emotions, fears, guilt and resentment. Have a professional help you prepare and be present during the Intervention. There is so much at stake in the Intervention that it is important to be well prepared and focused.

2. Select the Intervention team.

3. Learn about the process of Intervention with the help of your professional counselor. Watch a video of a dramatized Intervention to get the feel for it and whether you still want to be part of it.

4. Prepare, in writing, what you are going to say and determine the consequences you are going to present to the alcoholic if he or she does not enter treatment. Two powerful consequences are threat of divorce and the loss of a job. You must be prepared to follow through with your threat if the Intervention is to succeed.

5. Make arrangements for treatment. It is important that this is done before the Intervention so that the alcoholic can go directly to treatment from the Intervention — before he or she can think of any excuses why not to go!

6. Rehearse the Intervention. This allows for members of the Intervention team to rehearse what they are going to say in a group setting. It is important to remember that you are trying to offer your loved one a solution to their drinking. Express yourself with love and caring. The alcoholic thrives on confrontation. Love has the best shot of breaking resistance.

7. Do the Intervention. Having selected a time and place that will surprise your loved one and will have him or her as sober as possible, your loved one walks into a roomful of concerned people and the Intervention begins.

No matter how emotional the Intervention is, the alcoholic should not be allowed physical contact with any group member until he or she has agreed to enter treatment. If the Intervention proceeds without interruption, the last person to speak offers the options open to the alcoholic: be professionally evaluated at a treatment center and follow through with the recommendations from the evaluation or face the consequences that have been given.

H ow long does an Intervention take?

Interventions last approximately 30-60 minutes — when you have reached the goal of getting your loved one to agree to be evaluated at a treatment center or realize that you will not achieve the goal that day.

W hy does Intervention work?

Being surprised by a roomful of concerned people who express with love to what extent his or her drinking is affecting everybody, the alcoholic is moved to take action to stop the drinking. There is little room for arguing and the consequences offered (loss of family, job and anything else precious) do not seem too appealing! During the Intervention, the alcoholic finally realizes how his or her life is being affected by the drinking and that if help is not sought, alcohol may be all he or she has left.

W hat if the Intervention fails?

It cannot. The goal of getting the alcoholic to treatment may not have been reached but the secret is out. All involved in the Intervention have a new awareness and will not be able to play games any longer. No one around the alcoholic will be able to retreat into denial again.

Why don't more people do an Intervention?
Simply—they do not know about it! Or, how it works.

"Intervention can save a life, a family, a friendship."

It is common sense to take a method and try it.
If it fails, admit it frankly and try another.
But above all, try something.

Franklin D. Roosevelt

9

Treatment: The Types Of Help Available

"Reach out for help, not a drink."

A lcoholism is the most untreated treatable disease. It can be arrested permanently by not taking another drink.

There is help available to assist in the task of achieving sobriety. There are treatment centers opening up across the United States every day. There are more counsellors being trained in alcoholism each year. There are more doctors who have increased their knowledge of the disease of alcoholism. There are support groups starting daily around the United States. The Federal and State Governments are spending more on stopping the swelling tide of alcoholism—from information dissemination to treatment centers. There IS help out there.

Each person has different needs. Keep looking until you find a treatment program that suits you or a loved one. After all the pain and suffering that the alcoholism has already caused, it is worth spending the time to find the best treatment for you and a loved one.

What types of treatment are there available?

There are inpatient and outpatient facilities and community based support groups, the most well known and effective support group being Alcoholics Anonymous (AA).

Do all alcoholics have to be treated as an inpatient?

No, but it can improve the chances of recovery.

Many alcoholics, especially in the early stages, have found sobriety by just attending Alcoholics Anonymous or other support groups and many recovering alcoholics can be treated successfully as outpatients.

Others find that an inpatient setting provides the discipline in which to stop drinking and get the emotional, physical and spiritual support needed as they lose their "old friend" — drink.

Inpatient treatment is a must for those that are in need of medical attention, are in the late stages of the disease and need supervised withdrawal, and are in any way unable to care for themselves.

Are all treatment centers the same?

No. There are centers opening up all over the country in response to the growing awareness of alcoholism. Be very wary of any "quick cure" center. It is important to check the credentials of the center and make sure they have a program suited to your loved one's needs.

What should I look for in a treatment center's program?

It is advisable to select a program that:

1. Acknowledges that alcoholism is a disease, a disease that can be halted but not cured. Full recovery being dependent on total and continuous abstinence from alcohol or substitute drugs.

2. Educates the alcoholic and family about the disease of alcoholism and how to handle life without alcohol.

3. Has a staff that is experienced in the treatment of alcoholism.

4. Has nutrition as a part of treatment.

5. Has group counselling.

6. Involves the family in treatment and follow-up care.

7. Has thorough follow-up care.

8. Is preferably support-group oriented to assist in long-term sobriety.

Who will pay for the treatment?

Most insurance companies pay for treatment.

Alcoholics Anonymous and other support groups are free.

Why is total abstinence so important?

Alcoholics have no control over drinking. There is no such thing as "just one drink." For an alcoholic there is always the possibility of relapse. Although abstinence is demanding and requires constant attention, sobriety is easier for the alcoholic to achieve than any other solution.

D*o the family or I need to get any treatment?*

Yes. Alcoholism is a family disease and anyone who has lived with the alcoholic has been affected emotionally and psychologically. The family needs to get help at the same time as the alcoholic to prepare for the changes that will occur in a household of a recovering alcoholic. If the family gets help in changing its enabling behavior, there is less chance of the alcoholic having a relapse.

Your life has revolved around the drinking almost as much as the alcoholic's. If your loved one stops drinking, your life will alter too. Be prepared! Go to Al-Anon, other support groups or individual therapy. Even people who are not still living with the alcoholic have been affected and would be advised to get treatment.

W*hat is Alcoholics Anonymous (AA) and what are some of its principles?*

1. AA is a group of recovering alcoholics who help each other stay sober.

2. AA offers help to anyone with a drinking problem.

3. As all AA members are alcoholics, they have a special understanding of each other. AA provides ongoing help, advice and support.

4. AA encourages new members to stay off drink one day at a time which makes the task of maintaining sobriety easier. AA members learn to concentrate on avoiding only one drink: the first one.

5. In AA you are accepted for who you are, not what you do. You are all equal in AA.

6. AA allows you to keep your anonymity if that's what you want and does not ask you to join anything or sign anything.

7. AA is not a religious organization.

8. AA has groups all over the world which makes it easier for recovering alcoholics to travel knowing they can get support if needed.

9. AA has designed an effective 12-Step program to help in recovery.

10. AA is free and proven to be one of the most effective forms of treatment.

As with other forms of treatment, find an AA group that is best suited to your temperament and background and in which you feel most comfortable. Go to different groups for variety. Do what is best for your recovery.

A*re there other support groups besides Alcoholics Anonymous?*

Yes. There are other support groups that cater for the specialized needs of individuals and provide support for those that find AA is not for them. For example, two groups — Women for Sobriety and Rational Recovery — are growing in popularity.

W*hy is attending a support group important?*

Attending support group meetings greatly enhances the chances of the alcoholic remaining sober over an extended period. Support groups provide the ongoing follow-up care needed for staying sober and are readily accessible to every alcoholic. The knowledge that other people have gone through the same experiences as the alcoholic can be a strength and a comfort; the alcoholic is not alone.

C*an a relapse happen if the alcoholic has had treatment?*

Yes. Although the alcoholic is committed to recovery, he or she can still have a relapse. A relapse does not mean that the treatment has failed. Sometimes a relapse convinces the alcoholic that abstinence is the only way to handle the disease.

W*here do I find treatment centers and Alcoholics Anonymous?*

Turn to the next chapter and you will find addresses and telephone numbers for treatment centers and other help programs in your State.

You can also look in the telephone book under "alcoholism" for further listings and for your local Alcoholics Anonymous and Al-Anon groups.

Remember, alcoholism is a treatable disease. There is no need to suffer any more. Seek the help you or a loved one deserve. You are not alone. Recovery is possible.

Enjoy the journey to sobriety!

Good luck!

_____10

Where To Find Help

I f you or a loved one needs help you can contact one of the organizations or agencies listed below. Be cautious when selecting a facility or program. Ask questions; ask for referrals. Remember to keep looking until you find one best suited to your loved one's and your own needs.

The listings are divided into three sections:

NATIONAL RESOURCES

These include organizations that will give you general information, referral information, literature and support group information.

STATE AUTHORITIES

Your State Authority can refer you to a program, agency, organization or hospital that deals with alcohol abuse.

WHERE TO FIND HELP STATE BY STATE

You will find a selection of listings of organizations and agencies in towns and cities in your State. Many are referral agencies. If you would like a more comprehensive list of where to find help in a particular State, please send a self-addressed stamped envelope to: *Disa Publications, 350 Ward Avenue, Suite 106, Honolulu, HI 96814.* Disa Publications will send you a comprehensive list of the State/s you request.

NATIONAL RESOURCES

Al-Anon Family Group Headquarters
P.O. Box 862
Midtown Station
New York, NY 10018-0862
(212) 302-7240
Call or write to request information about meeting schedules in your area, for literature and other services offered. Alternately, look in your local telephone book for the Al-Anon in your area.

Alcoholics Anonymous
P.O. Box 459
Grand Central Station
New York, NY 10163-1100
Tel: (212) 686-1100
Call or write to request information about meeting schedules in your area, for literature and other services offered. Alternatively, look in your local telephone book for the Alcoholics Anonymous in your area.

The National Clearinghouse
For Alcohol And Drug Information
P.O. Box 2345
Rockville, MD 20847-2345
Tel: (800) 729-6686 or (301) 468-2600
An excellent and helpful source for information on various aspects of alcoholism. They offer advice over the phone and/or by mail.

The National Council On Alcoholism
and Drug Dependency
12 West 21st Street
New York, NY 10010
(800) NCA-CALL
(212) 206-6770
They are another major source of information on alcoholism and have local Council offices in all major cities.

STATE AUTHORITIES

Alabama

Division of Substance Abuse Services
200 Interstate Park Drive
P.O. Box 3710
Montgomery, AL 36193
(205) 270-4650

Alaska

Division of Alcoholism & Drug Abuse
P.O. Box 110607
Juneau, AK 99811-0607
(907) 465-2071

Arizona

Office of Substance Abuse
2122 East Highland
Phoenix, AZ 85016
(602) 381-8996

Arkansas

Bureau of Alcohol &
 Drug Abuse Prevention
108 E. 7th Street
400 Waldon Building
Little Rock, AR 72201
(501) 682-6650

California

Governor's Policy Council on
 Drug & Alcohol Abuse
1700 K Street, 5th Floor
Sacramento, CA 95814-4037
(916) 445-1943

Colorado

Alcohol & Drug Abuse Division
4300 Cherry Creek Drive, South
Denver, CO 80222-1530
(303) 692-2930

Connecticut

Department of Public Health &
 Addiction Services
999 Asylum Avenue, 3rd Floor
Hartford, CT 06105
(203) 566-4145

Delaware

Division of Alcoholism, Drug
 Abuse & Mental Health
1901 North DuPont Highway
Newcastle, DE 19720
(302) 577-4461

District of Columbia

DC Alcohol & Drug Abuse
 Services Administration
1300 First Street, N.E., Suite 325
Washington, DC 20002
(202) 727-1762

Florida

Department of Health &
 Rehabilitative Services
1317 Winewood Blvd.
Building 6, Room 183
Tallahassee, FL 32301
(904) 488-0900

Georgia

Alcohol & Drug Services Section
2 Peachtree Street NE, 4th Floor
Atlanta, GA 30309
(404) 657-6400

Hawaii

Alcohol & Drug Abuse Division
P.O. Box 3378
Honolulu, HI 96801
(808) 586-3962

Idaho

Division of Family & Children
Services
450 West State Street, 3rd Floor
Boise, ID 83702
(208) 334-5935

Illinois

Department of Alcoholism &
Substance Abuse
222 South College, 2nd Floor
Springfield, IL 62704
(217) 785-9067

Indiana

Division of Mental Health
W-353, 402 W Washington Street
Indianapolis, IN 46204-2739
(317) 232-7816

Iowa

Division of Substance Abuse &
Health Promotion
Lucas State Office Building, 3rd Floor
Des Moines, IA 50319
(515) 281-4417

Kansas

Alcohol & Drug Abuse Services
Biddle Building
300 Southwest Oakley
Topeka, KS 66606-1861
(913) 296-3925

Kentucky

Division of Substance Abuse
275 East Main Street
Frankfort, KY 40621
(502) 564-2880

Louisiana

Office of Alcohol & Drug Abuse
1201 Capitol Access Road
P.O. Box 2790-BIN #18
Baton Rouge, LA 70821-2790
(504) 342-6717

Maine

Office of Substance Abuse
State House Station #159
24 Stone Street
Augusta, ME 04333-0159
(207) 287-6330

Maryland

State Alcohol & Drug Abuse
Administration
201 West Preston Street
Baltimore, MD 21201
(410) 225-6925

Massachusetts

Division of Substance Abuse Services
150 Tremont Street
Boston, MA 02111
(617) 727-7985

Michigan

Center for Substance Abuse Services
3423 N. Logan/M.L. King Jr. Blvd.
P.O. Box 30195
Lansing, MI 48909
(517) 335-8808

Minnesota

Chemical Dependency Program
Division
444 Lafayette Road
St. Paul, MN 55155-3823
(612) 296-4610

Mississippi

Division of Alcohol & Drug Abuse
Robert E. Lee State Building
11th Floor
Jackson, MS 39201
(601) 359-1288

Missouri

Division of Alcohol & Drug Abuse
1706 East Elm Street
Jefferson City, MO 65109
(314) 751-4942

Montana

Alcohol & Drug Abuse Division
1539 11th Avenue
Helena, MT 59601-1301
(406) 444-2827

Nebraska

Division of Alcohol & Drug Abuse
P.O. Box 94728
Lincoln, NE 68509-4728
(402) 471-2851

Nevada

Bureau of Alcohol & Drug Abuse
505 East King Street, Room 500
Carson City, NV 89710
(702) 687-4790

New Hampshire

Office of Alcohol & Drug Abuse
  Prevention
105 Pleasant Street
Concord, NH 03301
(603) 271-6119

New Jersey

Division of Alcoholism, Drug
  Abuse & Addiction Services
CN 362
Trenton, NJ 08625-0362
(609) 292-5760

New Mexico

Behavioral Health Services
  Division/SA
Harold Runnels Building
Room 3200 North
1190 Saint Francis Drive
Sante Fe, NM 87501
(505) 827-2601

New York

Office of Alcoholism & Substance
  Abuse Services
Executive Park South
P.O. Box 8200
Albany, NY 12203
(518) 457-2061

North Carolina

Alcohol & Drug Services
325 North Salisbury Street
Raleigh, NC 27611
(919) 733-4670

North Dakota

Division of Alcoholism & Drug Abuse
Professional Building
1839 East Capitol Avenue
Bismarck, ND 58501
(701) 224-2769

Ohio

Department of Alcohol & Drug
  Addiction Services
Two Nationwide Plaza, 12th Floor
280 N. High Street
Columbus, OH 43215-2537
(614) 466-3445

Oklahoma

Substance Abuse Services
P.O. Box 53277, Capitol Station
Oklahoma City, OK 73152-3277
(405) 271-8653

Oregon

Office of Alcohol & Drug Abuse
 Programs
1178 Chemeketa Street, NE
Room 102
Salem, OR 97310
(503) 378-2163

Pennsylvania

Office of Drug & Alcohol Programs
P.O. Box 90
Harrisburg, PA 17108
(717) 787-9857

Rhode Island

Office of Substance Abuse
P.O. Box 20363
Cranston, RI 02920
(401) 464-2091

South Carolina

Commission on Alcohol &
 Drug Abuse
3700 Forest Drive
Columbia, SC 29204
(803) 734-9527

South Dakota

Division of Alcohol & Drug Abuse
Hillsview Plaza, East Hwy. 34
500 East Capitol
Pierre, SD 57501-5090
(605) 773-3123

Tennessee

Bureau of Alcohol & Drug
 Abuse Services
Cordell Hull Building, Room 255
Nashville, TN 37247-4401
(615) 741-1921

Texas

Commission on Alcohol &
 Drug Abuse
720 Brazos Street, Suite 403
Austin, TX 78701
(512) 867-8802

Utah

Division of Substance Abuse
120 North 200 West, 4th Floor
P.O. Box 45500
Salt Lake City, UT 84404
(801) 538-3939

Vermont

Office of Alcohol & Drug
 Abuse Programs
103 South Main Street
Waterbury, VT 05676
(802) 241-2170

Virginia

Office of Substance Abuse Services
109 Governor Street
P.O. Box 1797
Richmond, VA 23214
(804) 786-3906

Washington

Division of Alcohol &
 Substance Abuse
P.O. Box 45330
Olympia, WA 98504-5330
(206) 438-8200

West Virginia

Division of Alcoholism & Drug Abuse
State Capitol Complex
1900 Kanawha Blvd.
Building 6, Room B-738
Charleston, WV 25305
(304) 558-2276

Wisconsin

Bureau of Substance Abuse Services
1 West Wilson Street
P.O. Box 7851
Madison, WI 53707
(608) 266-3719

Wyoming

Wyoming Division Of
  Behavioral Health
447 Hathaway Building
Cheyenne, WY 82002
(307) 777-6494

Where To Find Help State By State

ALABAMA

Birmingham

Alcohol & Drug Abuse Council
1923 14th Avenue South
Birmingham, AL 35205
(205) 933-1213

Family & Child Services
3600 8th Avenue South
Suite W-102
Birmingham, AL 35222
(205) 324-3411

Univ of Alabama in Birmingham
UAB Substance Abuse Programs
3015 7th Avenue South
Birmingham, AL 35233
(205) 934-2118
Hotline: (800) 762-3790

Cullman

North Central Alabama
Substance Abuse Council
Cullmam County Courthouse
Cullman, AL 35055
(205) 739-3530

Gadsen

The Bridge Inc.
3232 Lay Springs Road
Route 3
Gadsen, AL 35901
(205) 546-6324

Jasper

Northwest Alabama Mental
  Health Center
1100 7th Avenue
Jasper, AL 35501
(205) 387-0541
Hotline: (800) 489-3971

Mobile

Mobile Mental Health Center Inc
2400 Gordon Smith Drive
Mobile, AL 36617
(205) 473-4423

Montgomery

Council on Substance Abuse/
  NCADD
415 South McDonough Street
Montgomery, AL 36104
(205) 262-7401
Hotline: (800) SOB-ER90

Phenix City

Phenix Medical Park Hospital
Genesis Center
1707 21st Avenue
Phenix City, AL 36868
(205) 291-8399
Hotline: (800) 741-4293

Tuscaloosa

Indian Rivers Mental Health Center
505 19th Avenue
Tuscaloosa, AL 35401
(205) 391-0118
Hotline: (205) 345-1600

Warrior

Parkside Lodge of Birmingham
1189 Allbritton Road
Warrior, AL 35180
(205) 647-1945
Hotline: (800) 648-1945

ALASKA

Anchorage

Alaska Council on the Prevention
of Alcohol & Drug Abuse Inc.
3333 Denali Street
Suite 201
Anchorage, AK 99503
(907) 258-6021
Hotline: (800) 478-7738

Charter North Hospital &
Counseling Centers
2530 Debarr Road
Anchorage, AK 99508
(907) 258-7575
Hotline: (800) 478-7575

North Star Adolescent Hospital
1650 South Bragaw Street
Anchorage, AK 99508
(907) 277-1522
Hotline: (800) 478-5437

Fairbanks

Fairbanks Memorial Hospital
1650 Cowles Street
Fairbanks, AK 99701
(907) 452-8047

Fairbanks Native Association Inc.
3100 South Cushman Street
Fairbanks, AK 99701
(907) 452-6251

Kodiak

Kodiak Council on Alcoholism
Kodiak, AK 99615
(907) 486-3535

Nome

Northern Lights Recovery Center
5th Avenue & Division Street
Community Health Services Bldg
Nome, AK 99762
(907) 443-3344

Wasilla

Alaska Addiction Rehabilitation
Services Inc.
Nugens Ranch
3701 Palmer-Wasilla Highway
Wasilla, AK 99687
(907) 376-4534

ARIZONA

Flagstaff

The Guidance Center
518 North LeRoux Street
Flagstaff, AZ 86001
(602) 774-3351

Kingman

Mohave Mental Health Clinic
1750 Beverly Street
Kingman, AZ 86401
(602) 757-8111

Mesa

Centro de Amistad Inc.
734 East Broadway
Mesa, AZ 85204
(602) 833-0227

Phoenix

National Council on Alcoholism &
Drug Dependency
2701 North 16th Street
Phoenix, AZ 85006
(602) 264-6214

Saint Lukes Behavioral Health Center
1800 East Van Buren Street
Phoenix, AZ 85006
(602) 251-8484

Terros Inc.
711 East Missouri Street
Phoenix, AZ 85014
(602) 266-1100
Hotline: (800) 293-1749

Prescott

West Yavapai Guidance Clinic
505 South Cortez Street
Prescott, AZ 86301
(602) 445 -7730

Tuscon

Arizona Center for Clinical
  Management
Help on Call Crisis Line
Tuscon, AZ 85733
(602) 323-9373

Codac Counseling Center
2530 East Broadway
Tuscon, AZ 85716
(602) 327-4505

Cottonwood de Tuscon
4110 Sweetwater Drive
Tuscon, AZ 85745
(602) 743-0411
Hotline: (800) 877-4520

ARKANSAS

Benton

Counseling Clinic Inc.
307 East Servier Street
Benton, AR 72015
(501) 778-0404

Fort Smith

Gateway House Inc.
1715 Grand Avenue
Fort Smith, AR 72901
(501) 783-8849

Sparks Recovery Center
1311 South I Street
Fort Smith, AR 72901
(501) 441-5500

Jonesboro

Crowleys Ridge Development
  Council
520 West Monroe Street
Jonesboro, AR 72401
(501) 933-0033
Hotline: (800) 264-2535

Little Rock

Baptist Rehabilitation Institute
9601 Interstate 630 Exit 7
Little Rock, AR 72205
(501) 223-7507

CPC Pinnacle Pointe Hospital
11501 Financial Center Parkway
Little Rock, AR 72211
(501) 223-3322
Hotline: (800) 880-3322

Saint Vincent Medical Center
2 Saint Vincent Center
Little Rock, AR 722205
(501) 376-1200
Hotline: (800) 225-1112

Pine Bluff

Jefferson Regional Medical Center
First Step Chemical
  Dependency Unit
1515 West 42nd Avenue
Pine Bluff, AR 71603
(501) 534-2273
(800) 766-1843

Southeast Arkansas Mental
  Health Center
2500 Rike Drive
Pine Bluff, AR 71613
(501) 534-1834
(800) 272-2008

CALIFORNIA

Bakersfield

Family & Substance Abuse
 Counseling Agency
1680 20th Street
Bakersfield, CA 93301
(805) 323-6285

Burbank

New Way Foundation
207 North Victory Boulevard
Burbank, CA 91502
(818) 842-9416
Hotline: (818) 846-9771

Concord

Bi Bett Corporation
Shennum Center
2090 Commerce Center
Concord, CA 94520
(510) 676-2580

Costa Mesa

Starting Point of Orange County
350 West Bay Street
Costa Mesa, CA 92627
(714) 642-3505
Hotline: (800) 556-2273

El Monte

Mid Valley Alcohol Education Center
3430 Cogswell Road
El Monte, CA 91732
(818) 448-1097

Eureka

Saint Josephs Hospital
Family Recovery Services
2700 Dolbeer Street
Eureka, CA 95501
(707) 445-9251
Hotline: (800) 334-4774

Fremont

Fremont Recovery Center
37957 Fremont Boulevard
Fremont, CA 94536
(510) 792-4357

Fresno

Alcoholism & Drug Abuse Council
1651 L Street
Fresno, CA 93721
(209) 266-9888

Hayward

Kaiser Permanente Medical Center
27400 Hesperian Boulevard
Hayward, CA 94545
(510) 784-4072
Hotline: 784-4080

Laguna Beach

South Coast Medical Center
31872 Coast Highway
Laguna Beach, CA 92677
(714) 499-7150

Long Beach

Charter Hospital of Long Beach
6060 Paramount Boulevard
Long Beach, CA 90805
(310) 220-1000
Hotline: (800) 262-1414

Phoenix Family Treatment Center
3620 Long Beach Boulevard
Long Beach, CA 90807
(310) 595-0328
Hotline: (800) 696-6628

Los Angeles

Alcohol & Drug Program
 Administration
714 West Olympic Boulevard
Los Angeles, CA 90015
(213) 624-3784
Hotline: (800) 564-6600

Covenant House
1325 North Western Avenue
Los Angeles, CA 90027
(213) 461-3131
Hotline: (800) 999-9999

National Council on Alcoholism &
  Drug Dependency/Los Angeles
600 South New Hampshire Avenue
Los Angeles, CA 90015
(213) 384-0403
Hotline: (800) 433-0416

Volunteers of America of Los Angeles
Alcohol Services
515 East 6th Street
Los Angeles, CA 90021
(213) 627-8002

Modesto

Stanislaus County Department of
  Mental Health
Alcohol Treatment Program
800 Scenic Drive
Modesto, CA 95350
(209) 525-6243

Oakland

West Oakland Health Center
1531 Jefferson Street
Oakland, CA 94607
(510) 271-8080
Hotline: 271-8089

Pasadena

Pasadena Council on Alcoholism
  & Drug Dependency
131 North El Molino Drive
Suite 320
Pasadena, CA 91101
(818) 795-9127

Pomona

American Hospital
  Substance Abuse Services
2180 West Valley Boulevard
Pomona, CA 91768
(714) 865-2336
Hotline: (800) 255-5483

Riverside

Community Behavioral Health
  Group Inc.
5995 Brockton Avenue
Riverside, CA 92506
(909) 784-3050

Sacramento

Family Service Center
8912 Volunteer Lane
Sacramento, CA 95826
(916) 368-3080

National Council on Alcoholism &
  Drug Dependency
650 Home Avenue
Sacramento, CA 95825
(916) 922-9217

Sutter Outpatient Drug &
  Alcohol Program
7700 Folsom Boulevard
Sacramento, CA 95826
(916) 386-3031
Hotline: (916) 386-3077

Salinas

Monterey County Health
  Department
140 West Gabilan Street
Salinas, CA 93901
(408) 755-5430

San Diego

Counseling & Recovery Institute
3233 3rd Avenue
San Diego, CA 92301
(619) 543-0333

Kaiser Permanente Medical Group
Chemical Dependency
  Recovery Unit
328 Maple Street
San Diego, CA 92103
(619) 696-3037

MCC Managed Behavioral
  Care Of California
9040 Friars Road
San Diego, CA 92108
(619) 521-2150
Hotline: (800) 866-6534

The Palavra Tree
1212 South 43rd Street
San Diego, CA 92113
(619) 263-7768

San Francisco

Freedom From Alcohol & Drugs
1353 48th Avenue
San Francisco, CA 94122
(415) 665-8077
Hotline: 665-9323

National Council on Alcoholism &
  Drug Addictions
944 Market Street
San Francisco, CA 94102
(415) 296-9900

Presidio Counseling Center
Cnr Maudlin & MacDonald Streets
Presidio/San Francisco Building 910
San Francisco, CA 94129
(415) 561-5470
Hotline: (415) 561-2485

San Francisco General Hospital
Tom Smith Substance Abuse Center
1001 Potrero Avenue
San Francisco, CA 94110
(415) 206-8091

San Jose

Justice Services
614 Tully Road
San Jose, CA 95111
(408) 299-7280

National Council on Alcoholism &
  Drug Dependency
1922 The Alameda
San Jose, CA 95126
(408) 241-5577
Hotline: (408) 267-4357

San Pedro

Beacon House Association
1003 South Beacon Street
San Pedro, CA 90731
(310) 514-4940

Santa Ana

MCC Managed Behavioral Care of
  California
1551 North Tustin Avenue
Santa Ana, CA 92701
(714) 479-1333
Hotline: (800) 879-9823

Santa Barbara

Council on Alcohol & Drug Abuse
133 East Haley Street
Santa Barbara, CA 93102
(805) 962-6195

Santa Cruz

Community Counseling Center
271 Water Street
Santa Cruz, CA 95060
(408) 423-2003

Santa Rosa

Sonoma County Alcohol Services
2759 Bennett Valley Road
Santa Rosa, CA 95404
(707) 528-4141

Stockton

Alcohol Recovery Center
7273 Murray Drive
Stockton, CA 95210
(209) 953-8210

Ventura ──────────────

Medical Support Services To
Substance Abusers
3291 Loma Vista Road
Ventura, CA 93003
(805) 652-6235

COLORADO

Boulder ──────────────

Boulder County Health Department
3450 Broadway
Boulder, CO 80304
(303) 441-1279
Hotline: (303) 441-1281

Colorado Springs──────────

McMaster Center For Alcohol &
  Drug Treatment
301 South Union Boulevard
Colorado Springs, CO 80910
(719) 578-3150

The Ark Inc.
423 South Cascade Street
Colorado Springs, CO 80903
(719) 520-9988
Hotline: (719) 684-9483

Denver ──────────────

Alcohol Counseling Services Of
  Colorado Inc.
1300 South Lafayette Street
Denver, CO 80210
(303) 777-8648

Community Alcohol/Drug
  Rehabilitation & Education Center
3315 Gilpin Street
Denver, CO 80205
(303) 295-2521
Hotline: (303) 792-9922

Porter Center For Behavioral Health
2525 South Downing Street
Denver, CO 80210
(303) 778-5774

Substance Treatment Services
320 West 8th Avenue
Denver, CO 80204
(303) 436-5690

Fort Collins ──────────────

New Beginnings
1225 Redwood Street
Fort Collins, CO 80524
(303) 493-3389
Hotline: (800) 950-5150

Pueblo ──────────────

ADAPCP Counseling Center
Pueblo Depot Activity
SDSTE-PU-ADCO
Pueblo, CO 81001
(719) 549-4402

CONNECTICUT

Bridgeport──────────────

Chemical Abuse Services Agency Inc
690 Artic Street
Bridgeport, CT 06604
(203) 333-3887

Southern CT Mental Health &
  Substance Abuse Treatment Center
4920 Main Street
Bridgeport, CT 06606
(203) 365-8400
Hotline: (203) 254-2000

Hartford──────────────

Alcohol & Drug Recovery
  Centers Inc.
500 Vine Street
Hartford, CT 06112
(203) 243-8931

Regional Alcohol & Drug Abuse
Resources Inc.
645 Farmington Avenue
Hartford, CT 06105
(203) 523-9788

Middletown

The Connection Inc.
Greater Middletown Counseling
Center
196 Court Street
Middletown, CT 06457
(203) 343-5510

New Haven

Affiliates For Consultation & Therapy
389 Orange Street
New Haven, CT 06511
(203) 562-4235

Alcohol Treatment Unit
285 Orchard Street
New Haven, CT 06511
(203) 789-7387

New London

Care Center
516 Vauxhall Street
New London, CT 06320
(203) 442-3380

Stamford

Alcohol & Drug Abuse Council
159 Colonial Road
Stamford, CT 06906
(203) 325-1511

Liberations Programs Inc.
119 Main Street
Stamford, CT 06901
(203) 359-3134

Waterbury

Family Intervention Center
1875 Thomaston Avenue
Waterbury, CT 06704
(203) 753-2153

Morris Foundation
142 Griggs Street
Waterbury, CT 06704
(203) 574-3986

DELAWARE

Dover

Because We Care II
48A McKee Road
Dover, DE 19901
(302) 734-2301

Wilmington

A & D Associates
5211 West Woodmill Drive
Wilmington, DE 19808
(302) 998-8771

Family & Children Services
2005 Baynard Boulevard
Wilmington, DE 19802
(302) 658-5177

New Beginnings
5205 West Woodmill Drive
Wilmington, DE 19808
(302) 995-2124
Hotline: (800) 365-1919

People's Settlement
408 East 8th Street
Wilmington, DE 19801
(302) 658-4133
Hotline: (302) 657-2851

DISTRICT OF COLUMBIA

A L Nellum & Associates Inc.
2700 Martin Luther King Avenue SE
Saint Elizabeth Hospital Building N
Washington, DC 20036
(202) 466-4920

Center For Child Protection &
  Family Support
714 G Street SE
Washington, DC 20036
(202) 544-3144

Concerned Citizens On Alcohol &
  Drug Abuse
3115 Martin Luther King Avenue SE
Washington, DC 20007
(202) 338-0654

Georgetown University
Alcohol & Drug Abuse Program
3800 Reservoir Road NW
Washington, DC 20007
(202) 687-8770

Project Care
415 Edgewood Street NE
Suite B-3
Washington, DC 20017
(202) 635-CARE

Council On Alcoholism &
  Drug Abuse Inc.
2813 12th Street NE
Washington, DC 20017
(202) 526-0975
Hotline: (202) 783-1300

FLORIDA

Boca Raton

National Recovery Institute
1000 NW 15th Street
Boca Raton, FL 33486
(407) 392-8444
Hotline: (800) 535-5844

Clearwater

Family Resources Inc.
626 Lakeview road
Clearwater, FL 34616
(813) 461-1424
Hotline: (813) 531-4664

Daytona Beach

Atlantic Treatment Center Inc.
841 Jimmy Ann Drive
Daytona Beach, FL 32117
(904) 274-5333
Hotline: (800) 345-2647

Pioneer Healthcare Inc.
433 Silver Beach Avenue
Daytona Beach, FL 32118
(904) 253-8681
Hotline: (800) 821-4357

Delray Beach

Drug Abuse Foundation Of
  Palm Beach
400 South Swinton Avenue
Delray Beach, FL 33444
(407) 278-0000

Fort Lauderdale

Alternative Substance Abuse
  Systems Inc.
613 SE First Avenue
Fort Lauderdale, FL 33301
(305) 462-2005

Court Alcohol & Substance
  Abuse Program
624 SW First Avenue
Fort Lauderdale, FL 33301
(305) 763-4505

Fort Myers

Charter Glade Hospital
Chemical Dependency Unit
3550 Colonial Boulevard
Fort Myers, FL 33906
(813) 939-0403
Hotline: (800) 274-1230

Fort Pierce

Drug Abuse Treatment
  Association Inc.
4590 Selvitz Road
Fort Pierce, FL 34981
(407) 465-4050

Gainesville

Charter Counseling Center
611 NW 60th Street
Gainesville, FL 32607
(904) 331-8559
Hotline: (800) 334-1455

Jacksonville

Gateway Community Services Inc.
555 Stockton Street
Jacksonville, FL 32204
(904) 387-4661

Next Step
6428 Beach Boulevard
Jacksonville, FL 32216
(904) 724-9373
Hotline: (904) 724-6500

River Region Human Services Inc.
3728 Philips Highway
Jacksonville, FL 32207
(904) 348-0919
Hotline: (904) 359-6577

Key West

Lower Florida Keys Health
  System Inc.
1200 Kennedy Drive
Key West, FL 33040
(305) 294-5531
Hotline: (800) 233-3119

Miami

Bayview Centers Inc.
9325 Park Drive
Miami, FL 33138
(305) 751-5700

Community Health Of South Dade
Substance Abuse Services
10300 SW 216th Street
Miami, FL 33190
(305) 252-4848
Hotline: (305) 255-1850

Kedem Counseling Center Inc.
5730 Bird Road
Miami, FL 33155
(305) 447-1050
Hotline: (305) 323-6070

Metro Dade Department Of
  Human Resources
111 NW First Street
Miami, FL 33128
(305) 375-5750
Hotline: (305) 638-6540

The Village South Inc.
400 NE 31st Street
Miami, FL 33137
(305) 573-3784
Hotline: (800) 433-3784

Naples

David Lawrence Center
6075 Golden Gate Parkway
Naples, FL 33999
(813) 649-1404
Hotline: (813) 455-4376

Ocala

Comp Addiction Treatment Services
2105 SW College Road
Ocala, FL 32674
(904) 732-2287

Orlando

Center For Drug Free Living Inc.
100 West Columbia Street
Orlando, FL 32806
(407) 423-6618

Colonial Counseling Associates
1400 Hillcrest Street
Orlando, FL 32803
(407) 895-3580

Substance Abuse Family Education
2400 Silver Star Road
Orlando, FL 32804
(407) 291-4357

Pensacola

Community Alcohol &
  Drug Commission
803 North Palafox Street
Pensacola, FL 32501
(904) 434-2724

Saint Petersburg

Family Resources Inc.
5235 16th Street North
Saint Petersburg, FL 33733
(813) 526-1100
Hotline: (813) 521-4664

MCC Behavioral Care Inc.
888 Executive Center Drive West
Saint Petersburg, FL 33702
(813) 577-9088
Hotline: (800) 274-4573

Sarasota

Sarasota Memorial New Dawn
  Center For Alcohol &
  Drug Treatment
1700 South Tamiami Trail
Sarasota, FL 34239
(813) 953-1783

Tallahassee

A Life Recovery Center
1212 South Monroe Street
Tallahassee, FL 32301
(904) 224-9991
Hotline: (800) 755-9981

Tampa

Agency For Community
  Treatment Services Inc.
4211 East Busch Boulevard
Tampa, Florida 33617
(813) 988-6096

Florida Counseling Inc.
5401 West Kennedy Boulevard
Tampa, FL 33609
(813) 289-3396
Hotline: (813) 289-3272

West Palm Beach

Hanley Hazelden Center At
  Saint Marys
5200 East Avenue
West Palm Beach, FL 33407
(407) 848-1666
Hotline: (800) 444-7008

GEORGIA

Atlanta

Dekalb Addiction Clinic
1260 Briarcliff Road NE
Atlanta, GA 30306
(404) 894-5808
Hotline: (404) 892-4646

Fulton County Drug &
  Alcohol Treatment Center
265 Boulevard Street NE
Atlanta, GA 30312
(404) 730-1616

Augusta

CMHC Of East Central Georgia
Alcohol & Drug Services
3421 Old Savannah Road
Augusta, GA 30906
(706) 771-4800
Hotline: (706) 560-2943

Columbus

Alcohol & Drug Services
1334 2nd Avenue
Columbus, GA 31901
(404) 324-3701
Hotline: (706) 327-3999

Dalton

Hamilton Medical Center
Burleyson Drive
Dalton, GA 30720
(706) 272-6480
Hotline: (800) 441-6480

Decatur

Fox Recovery Center
3100 Clifton Springs Road
Decatur, GA 30034
(404) 241-8063
Hotline: (404) 892-4646

Dublin

Middle Georgia Alcohol &
  Drug Clinic
600 North Jefferson Street
Dublin, GA 31021
(912) 275-6800
Hotline: (912) 275-6810

Griffin

McIntosh Trail MH/MR/SA Services
1459 Williamson Road
Griffin, GA 30223
(404) 229-3158
Hotline: (800) 282-1120

Macon

Crisis Stabilization Program
3575 Fulton Mill Road
Macon, GA 31206
(912) 741-8113

Valdosta

Greenleaf Center Inc.
2209 Pineview Drive
Valdosta, GA 31602
(912) 247-4357
Hotline: (800) 247-2747

HAWAII

Hilo

Big Island Substance Abuse Council
1190 Waianuenue Avenue
Hilo, HI 96721
(808) 935-4927
Hotline: (808) 935-4972

Honolulu

Coalition For A Drug Free Hawaii
1218 Waimanu Street
Honolulu, HI 96814
(808) 524-1111

Drug Addiction Services Of Hawaii
1031 Auahi Street
Honolulu, HI 96814
(808) 523-0704
Hotline: (808) 523-0400

Kailua

Hawaii Counseling &
  Education Center Inc.
970 North Kalaheo Avenue
Kailua, HI 96734
(808) 254-6484

Lihue

Kauai Outreach Program
4444 Rice Street
Lihue, HI 96766
(808) 245-5959

Waianae

Waianae Coast Community
  MH Center
85-670 Farrington Highway
Waianae, HI 96792
(808) 696-4211

Wailuku

Maui Youth & Family Services
16 South Market Street
Wailuku, HI 96793
(808) 242-4757
Hotline: (808) 579-8406

IDAHO

Boise ———————

Alcoholism Intervention Services
8436 Fairview Avenue
Boise, ID 83704
(208) 322-8046

Care Institute
4696 Overland Street
Boise, ID 83705
(208) 384-1944
Hotline: (800) 974-0118

CPC Intermountain Hospital
Of Boise
303 North Allumbaugh Street
Boise, ID 83704
(208) 377-8400

Northwest Passages &
Counseling Center
131 North Allumbaugh Street
Boise, ID 83704
(208) 322-5922
Hotline: (800) 634-2638

Idaho Falls ———————

Aspen Crest Counseling Center
1970 East 17th Street
Idaho Falls, ID 83404
(208) 523-4072
Hotline: (800) 423-3710

Nampa ———————

Care Institute
508 East Florida Street
Nampa, ID 83686
(208) 463-0118
Hotline: (800) 974-0118

Pocatello ———————

Aspen Crest Counseling Center
797 Hospital Way
Pocatello, ID 83201
(208) 234-0797
Hotline: (800) 423-3710

ILLINOIS

Aurora ———————

Community Counseling Center
Of Fox Valley Inc.
479 North Lake Street
Aurora, IL 60505
(708) 897-0584

Chicago ———————

Alternatives Inc.
1126 West Granville Avenue
Chicago, IL 60660
(312) 973-5400

Cook County Hospital
1835 West Harrison Street
B Building, 2nd Floor
Chicago, IL 60612
(312) 633-5684

Human Resources
Development Institute
417 South Dearborn Street
Chicago, IL 60608
(312) 226-6989

Interventions
1234 South Michigan Avenue
Chicago, IL 60605
(312) 663-1020
Hotline: (312) 239-2370

Southeast Alcohol & Drug
Abuse Center
9101 South Exchange Avenue
Chicago, IL 60617
(312) 731-9100

Substance Abuse Services Inc.
2101 South Indiana Avenue
Chicago, IL 60616
(312) 808-3210

Danville

Crosspoint Human Services
309 North Logan Avenue
Danville, IL 61832
(217) 442-3200

Decatur

Decatur Mental Health Center
403 Longview Place
Decatur, IL 62521
(217) 422-3325

Freeport

Martin Luther King Jr.
 Community Services
511 South Liberty Street
Freeport, IL 61032
(815) 233-9915

Jacksonville

The Wells Center
1300 Lincoln Avenue
Jacksonville, IL 62650
(217) 243-1871

Joliet

Silver Cross Hospital
Chemical Dependency Unit
1200 Maple Road
Joliet, IL 60432
(815) 740-7034
Hotline: (815) 740-7039

Kankakee

Parkside Lodge South
401 North Wall Street
Kankakee, IL 60901
(815) 935-1844
Hotline: (800) 465-3565

Maywood

Youth Outreach Services Inc.
1701 South First Avenue
Maywood, IL 60153
(708) 343-5900

Peoria

Human Service Center
3400 New Leaf Lane
Peoria, IL 61615
(309) 692-6900

Quincy

Saint Mary Hospital Behavioral
 Health Services
1415 Vermont Street
Quincy, IL 62301
(217) 223-1200
Hotline: (800) 222-9413

Rock Island

Robert Young Center For
 Community Mental Health
2701 17th Street
Rock Island, IL 61201
(309) 793-3000
Hotline: (800) 322-1431

Rockford

Addiction Treatment &
 Education Program
5758 Elaine Drive
Rockford, IL 61108
(815) 229-3233
Hotline: (815) 961-6000

Skokie

Northern Illinois Counseling
 Services Inc.
9933 North Lawler Street
Skokie, IL 60077
(708) 676-0113

Springfield

Saint Johns Hospital Libertas
 Program
800 East Carpenter Street
Springfield, IL 62769
(217) 525-5629

Waterloo

Human Support Services Of
  Monroe County
988 North Market Street
Waterloo, IL 62298
(618) 939-8644
(618) 251-4073 A/H

Waukegan

Lake County Health Department
2400 Belvidere Street
Waukegan, IL 60085
(708) 360-6540
Hotline: (708) 872-4242

Wheaton

Du Page County Health Department
111 North County Farm Road
Wheaton, IL 60187
(708) 682-7560
Hotline: (708) 622-1700

Woodstock

Memorial Hospital For
  McHenry County
527 West South Street
Woodstock, IL 60098
(815) 338-2500
Hotline: (800) 675-8448

INDIANA

Anderson

Crestview Center
2201 Hillcrest Drive
Anderson, IN 46012
(317) 649-1961
Hotline: (317) 649-4357

Bloomington

Argo Counseling Inc.
118 East 6th Street
Bloomington, IN 47408
(812) 331-1033

Bloomington Meadows Hospital
3800 North Prow Road
Bloomington, IN 47404
(812) 331-8000
Hotline: (800) 972-4410

Elkhart

Elkhart General Hospital
600 East Boulevard
Elkhart, IN 46515
(219) 523-3370
Hotline: (800) 274-5433

Evansville

Deaconess Hospital
600 Mary Street
Evansville, IN 47747
(812) 426-3496
Hotline: (800) 467-4174

Fort Wayne

Charter Beacon Hospital
1720 Beacon Street
Fort Wayne, IN 46805
(219) 423-3651
Hotline: (800) 462-7491

Gary

Southlake Center For Mental
  Health Inc.
8555 Taft Street
Gary, IN 46410
(219) 769-4005

Indianapolis

Charter Counseling Centers
5663 Caito Drive
Indianapolis, IN 46226
(317) 547-1800
Hotline: (800) 843-9299

Family Service Association
615 North Alabama Street
Indianapolis, IN 46204
(317) 634-6341

Midwest Medical Center
3232 North Meridian Street
Indianapolis, IN 46208
(317) 924-3392

Kokomo

Saint Joseph Hospital
1907 West Sycamore Street
Kokomo, IN 46902
(317) 459-5187

Lafayette

Family Services Inc.
731 Main Street
Lafayette, IN 47901
(317) 423-5361

South Bend

Madison Center Inc.
403 East Madison Street
South Bend, IN 46601
(219) 234-0061

Terra Haute

Hamilton Center Inc.
620 8th Avenue
Terra Haute, IN 47804
(812) 231-8281
Hotline: (800) 742-0787

Valparaiso

Porter/Starke CMHC
  Substance Abuse Services
701 Wall Street
Valparaiso, IN 46383
(219) 464-8541

IOWA

Ames

Center For Addictions Recovery
511 Duff Avenue
Ames, IA 50010
(515) 232-3206

Burlington

Burlington Medical Center
602 North 3rd Street
Burlington, IA 52601
(319) 753-3633

Cedar Rapids

Foundation II Inc.
1540 2nd Avenue SE
Cedar Rapids, IA 52403
(319) 362-2174
(800) 332-4224

Davenport

Center For Alcohol & Drug Services
1523 South Fairmount Street
Davenport, IA 52802
(319) 322-2667

Des Moines

Children & Families Of Iowa
1111 University Street
Des Moines, IA 50314
(515) 288-1981

Harold Hughes Centers
600 East 14th Street
Des Moines, IA 50316
(515) 265-3400
Hotline: (800) 247-0764

Iowa City

Mid Eastern Council On
  Chemical Abuse
430 Southgate Avenue
Iowa City, IA 52240
(319) 351-4357

Ottumwa

Family Recovery Center
312 East Alta Vista Avenue
Ottumwa, IA 52501
(515) 684-4651
(800) 933-6742

Sioux City

Saint Lukes Gordon Recovery
  Centers
2720 Stone Park Boulevard
Sioux City, IA 51104
(712) 279-3960
Hotline: (800) 472-9018

Spirit Lake

Northwest Iowa Alcoholism &
  Drug Treatment Unit Inc.
Dickinson County Memorial Hospital
Spirit Lake, IA 51360
(712) 336-4560

KANSAS

Emporia

Mental Health Center Of East
  Central Kansas
1000 Lincoln Street
Emporia, KS 66801
(316) 342-0548

Garden City

Western Kansas Foundation
  For Alcoholism & Drug
  Dependency Inc.
811 North Main Street
Garden City, KS 67846
(316) 275-7103

Great Bend

Center For Counseling &
  Consultation
5815 Broadway
Great Bend, KS 67530
(316) 792-2544

Hays

Key Alcohol & Drug Abuse Services
1008 East 17th Street
Hays, KS 67601
(913) 628-2240

Kansas City

Heart Of America Family
  Services Inc.
5424 State Avenue
Kansas City, KS 66102
(913) 287-1300

Kansas City Drug & Alcohol
  Information School
707 Minnesota Avenue
Kansas City, KS 66101
(913) 342-3011

Manhattan

Northeast Kansas Regional
  Prevention Center
2001 Claflin Street
Manhattan, KS 66502
(913) 587-4372

Newton

Prairie View Mental Health Center
1901 East First Street
Newton, KS 67114
(316) 283-2400
Hotline : (800) 362-0810

Overland Park

Heart Of America Family
  Services Inc.
10500 Barkley Street
Overland Park, KS 66212
(913) 642-4300

Shawnee Mission

Alcohol & Drug Services Inc.
6005 Martway Street
Shawnee Mission, KS 66202
(913) 722-3866

Topeka

National Council On Alcoholism
603 SW Topeka Boulevard
Topeka, KS 66603
(913) 235-8622

Sunflower Alcohol Safety Action
  Project Inc.
112 SE 7th Street
Topeka, KS 66603
(913) 232-1415

KENTUCKY

Ashland

Pathways Inc.
201 22nd Street
Ashland, KY 41101
(606) 324-1141
Hotline: (800) 562-8909

Bowling Green

Lifeskills Inc.
822 Woodway
Bowling Green, KY 42101
(502) 842-2696
Hotline: (800) 223-8913

Corbin

Baptist Regional Medical Center
  Chemical Dependency Unit
1 Trillium Way
Corbin, KY 40701
(606) 528-1212
Hotline: (800) 395-4435

Covington

Family Alcohol & Drug
  Counseling Center
722 Scott Street
Covington, KY 41012
(606) 431-2225

Frankfort

Bluegrass Education & Treatment
  Of Alcoholism Program
943 Wash Road
Frankfort, KY 40601
(502) 223-2017
Hotline: (800) 928-8000

Henderson

Regional Addiction Resources
6347 Highway 60 East
Henderson, KY 42420
(502) 827-8314
Hotline: (800) 433-7291

Lexington

Bluegrass East Comprehensive
  Care Center
200 West 2nd Street
Lexington, KY 40507
(606) 281-2100
Hotline: (800) 928-8000

Growth Resources
1517 Nicholasville Road
Lexington, KY 40503
(606) 276-1194
Hotline: (800) 928-8000

National Council On Alcoholism
629 North Broadway
Lexington, KY 40587
(606) 254-2761

Louisville

Frager Associates
3906 Du Pont Square South
Louisville, KY 40207
(502) 893-6654

Ten Broeck Hospital
Substance Abuse Services
8521 La Grange Road
Louisville, KY 40242
(502) 426-6380

Ultimate Care
10400 Linn Station Road
Louisville, KY 40223
(502) 339-8552

Newport

Comp Care Centers Of
  Northern Kentucky
10th & Monmouth Streets
Newport, KY 41071
(606) 431-4450

Paducah

Joseph Friedman Substance
  Abuse Center
1405 South 3rd Street
Paducah, KY 42003
(502) 442-9131
Hotline: (800) 592-3980

LOUISIANA

Alexandria

Crossroads Regional Hospital
110 John Eskew Drive
Alexandria, LA 71315
(318) 445-5111

Baton Rouge

Council Of Greater Baton Rouge
1801 Florida Boulevard
Baton Rouge, LA 70802
(504) 343-8330

Baton Rouge Substance Abuse Clinic
4615 Government Street
Baton Rouge, LA 70806
(504) 922-0050
Hotline: (504) 924-3900

CPC Meadowwood Hospital
Center For Addictive Disorders
9032 Perkins Road
Baton Rouge, LA 70810
(504) 766-8553

Lafayette

Lafayette Alcohol & Drug
  Abuse Clinic
400 Saint Julien Street
Lafayette, LA 70506
(318) 262-5870

Lake Charles

Charter Health Systems
4250 5th Avenue South
Lake Charles, LA 70605
(800) 234-9192
Hotline: (800) CHA-RTER

Monroe

Monroe Alcohol & Drug Abuse Clinic
3208 Concordia Street
Monroe, LA 71201
(318) 362-5188
Hotline: (318) 387-5683

New Orleans

Coliseum Medical Center
3601 Coliseum Street
New Orleans, LA 70115
(504) 897-9700
Hotline: (504) 899-5119

Family Service Of Greater
  New Orleans
2515 Canal Street
New Orleans, LA 70119
(504) 822-0800

The Velocity Foundation
1001 Howard Avenue
New Orleans, LA 70113
(504) 525-5463
Hotline: (504) 581-7143

Shreveport

Council On Alcoholism & Drug
  Abuse Of Northwest Louisiana
820 Jordan Street
Shreveport, LA 71101
(318) 222-8511

CPC Brentwood Hospital
Chemical Dependency Unit
1800 Irving Place
Shreveport, LA 71101
(318) 424-6761

First Step Services Inc.
2000 Creswell Street
Shreveport, LA 71104
(318) 222-4222

Thibodaux

Thibodaux Alcohol & Drug
  Abuse Clinic
303 Hickory Street
Thibodaux, LA 70301
(504) 447-0851
Hotline: (800) 622-4126

MAINE

Bangor

Alternative Counseling Services
263 State Street
Bangor, ME 04401
(207) 990-5002
Hotline: (207) 823-6946

Community Health &
  Counseling Services
42 Cedar Street
Bangor, ME 04401
(207) 947-0366

Northeast Care Foundation
257 Harlow Street
Bangor, ME 04401
(207) 924-5520

Lewiston

Harbor Light Associates
145 Lisbon Street
Lewiston, ME 04241
(207) 783-8968

Lincoln

Community Health &
  Counseling Services
Transalpine Road
Lincoln, ME 04457
(207) 794-3554

Portland

Smith House Inc.
91-93 State Street
Portland, ME 04101
(207) 772-8822

MARYLAND

Annapolis

Anne Arundel County
  Health Department
62 Cathedral Street
Annapolis, MD 21401
(410) 222-1244

Renewal & Recovery Center
  Of Annapolis
2525 Riva Road
Annapolis, MD 21401
(410) 224-3336
Hotline: (800) 756-3336

Baltimore

American Council On
  Alcoholism Inc.
5024 Campbell Boulevard
Baltimore, MD 21236
(410) 931-9393
Hotline: (800) 5275344

Baltimore City Health Department
4 South Frederick Street
Baltimore, MD 21202
(410) 396-1141

Family Service Foundation Inc.
4806 Seton Drive
Baltimore, MD 21215
(410) 764-0663

Mountain Manor Treatment Center
3800 Frederick Street
Baltimore, MD 21229
(410) 233-1400
Hotline: (800) 537-3422

Total Health Care Inc.
1609 Druid Hill Avenue
Baltimore, MD 21217
(301) 383-7711

Bel Air

Recovery With Dignity
2107 Laurel Bush Road
Bel Air, MD 21014
(410) 879-4488
Hotline: (410) 494-8123

Bethesda

Counseling Institute Of
  Suburban MD
4401 East West Highway
Bethesda, MD 20814
(301) 654-7021

College Park

Changing Point Health Services Inc.
10013 Rhode Island Avenue
College Park, MD 20740
(301) 345-9181
Hotline: (800) 883-5100

Ellicott City

Howard County Addictions
  Service Center
3545 Ellicott Mills Drive
Ellicott City, MD 21043
(410) 465-0127

Frederick

Frederick County Substance
  Abuse Services
350 Montvue Lane
Frederick, MD 21702
(301) 694-1778

Hagerstown

Addiction Specialist Associates
138 East Antietam Street
Hagerstown, MD 21740
(301) 739-3752
Hotline: (800) 877-3752

Laurel

Key Center For Human Services Inc.
300 Thomas Drive
Laurel, MD 20707
(301) 776-1814

Rockville

Another Path
14901 Broschart Road
Rockville, MD 20850
(301) 251-4525

Montgomery County Government
Substance Abuse Prevention
401 Fleet Street
Rockville, MD 20850
(301) 217-1107
Hotline: (301) 770-3280

Salisbury

New Beginnings
1202 Old Ocean City Road
Salisbury, MD 21801
(410) 548-2300

Silver Spring

Kolmac Clinic
1003 Spring Street
Silver Spring, MD 20910
(301) 589-0255

Westminster

Reentry Mental Health Services
40 South Church Street
Westminster, MD 21157
(410) 848-9244

MASSACHUSETTS

Boston

Bay Cove Human Services
104 Lincoln Street
Boston, MA 02111
(617) 350-6270

MSPCC Family Counseling Center
95 Berkeley Street
Boston, MA 02116
(617) 426-1055

Spaulding Rehabilitation Hospital
125 Nashua Street
Boston, MA 02114
(617) 720-6991
Hotline: (617) 720-6701

Addiction Treatment Center
Of NE INC.
77 Warren Street F
Boston, MA 02135
(617) 254-1271

First Inc./First Step
34 Intervale Street
Boston, MA 02121
(617) 445-5230
Hotline: (617) 445-1500

Peaceful Movement Committee Inc.
879 Blue Hill Avenue
Boston, MA 02124
(617) 436-3159

After Care Services
1A Monmouth Square
Boston, MA 02128
(617) 569-4561

Faulkner Hospital
1153 Center Street
Boston, MA 02130
(617) 983-7711

Dimock Community Health Center
55 Dimock Street
Boston, MA 02119
(617) 442-9686

South Boston Action Council Inc.
424 West Broadway
Boston, MA 02127
(617) 269-5160

Brockton

MSPCC Family Counseling Center
130 Liberty Street
Brockton, MA 02401
(508) 586-3290

Cambridge

Cambridge Hospital
1493 Cambridge Street
Cambridge, MA 02139
(617) 498-1420

Fall River

Family Service Association
Of Greater Fall River
151 Rock Street
Fall River, MA 02720
(508) 678-7541

Framingham

South Middlesex Addiction Services
63 Fountain Street
Framingham, MA 01701
(508) 879-6320

Gloucester

Greater Cape Ann Human
Services Mental Health Center
Addison Gilbert Hospital
298 Washington Street
Gloucester, MA 01930
(508) 283-0293
Hotline: (508) 283-4000

Holyhoke

Providence Hospital
317 Maple Street
Holyhoke, MA 01040
(413) 535-1000

Lawrence

Family Services Association
  Of Greater Lawrence
430 North Canal Street
Lawrence, MA 01840
(508) 683-9505

Lowell

Family Service Of Greater Lowell
97 Central Street
Lowell, MA 01852
(508) 937-3000

New Bedford

Center For Health & Human Services
800 Purchase Street
New Bedford, MA 02741
(508) 990-3126

Northampton

Cooley Dickinson Hospital
76 Pleasant Street
Northampton, MA 01060
(413) 586-8550

Pittsfield

Berkshire Council on Alcoholism
131 Bradford Street
Pittsfield, MA 01202
(413) 499-1000

Plymouth

National Alcoholism Programs
1233 State Street
Plymouth, MA 02360
(508) 224-7701

Quincy

Bay State Community Services Inc.
15 Cottage Avenue
Quincy, MA 02169
(617) 472-4649

Salem

Health & Education Services
162 Federal Street
Salem, MA 01970
(508) 745-2440

Somerville

Caspar Inc.
226 Highland Avenue
Somerville, MA 02143
(617) 623-2080

Springfield

Alcohol & Drug Services Of
  Western Massachusetts Inc.
1400 State Street
Springfield, MA 01109
(413) 736-0334

Waltham

Middlesex Human Service
  Agency Inc.
775 Trapelo Road
Waltham, MA 02254
(617) 894-6110

Worcester

Adcare Hospital
107 Lincoln Street
Worcester, MA 01605
(508) 799-9000
Hotline: (800) ALC-OHOL

MSPCC Family Counseling Center
286 Lincoln Street
Worcester, MA 01605
(508) 753-2967
Hotline: (800) 442-3035

MICHIGAN

Ann Arbor

Ann Arbor Community Center
625 North Main Street
Ann Arbor, MI 48104
(313) 662-3128

Occupational Health Centers
  Of America
3800 Packard Street
Ann Arbor, MI 48108
(313) 482-8900
Hotline: (800) 852-0357

Battle Creek

New Day Center Of Battle Creek
330 East Columbia Street
Battle Creek, MI 49016
(616) 964-7121
Hotline: (616) 962-9006

Bay City

Bay Haven Chemical Dependency
  & Mental Health Programs
713 9th Street
Bay City, MI 48708
(517) 894-3799
Hotline: (800) 526-7314

Birmingham

Evergreen Counseling Centers
999 Haynes Street
Birmingham, MI 48009
(313) 645-0432
Hotline: (800) 837-6424

Dearborn

Family Service Of Detroit/
  Wayne County
19855 West Outer Drive
Dearborn, MI 48124
(313) 274-5840
Hotline: (313) 863-0700

Detroit

Boniface Community Action
  Corporation
1025 East Forest Street
Detroit, MI 48201
(313) 577-9100

Family Service Of Detroit
220 Bagley Street
Detroit, MI 48226
(313) 965-2141
Hotline: (313) 863-0700

Health Service Technical
  Assistance Inc.
1545 East Lafayette Street
Detroit, MI 48207
(313) 259-6411

Michigan Health Center
2700 Martin Luther King Jr Blvd.
Detroit, MI 48208
(313) 863-8000
Hotline: (313) 755-0600

National Council On Alcoholism
  & Drug Dependency
10601 West Seven Mile Road
Detroit, MI 48221
(313) 861-0666

Neighborhood Service Organization
3430 3rd Street
Detroit, MI 48201
(313) 963-1525
Hotline: (313) 963-1555

Wayne State University
656 West Kirby Street
Faculty Administration
Building 3049
Detroit, MI 48202
(313) 577-8834

Farmington Hills

Farmington Area Advisory
  Council Inc.
23450 Middlebelt Road
Farmington Hills, MI 48336
(313) 477-6767

Flint

Insight Recovery Center Inc
1110 Eldon Baker Drive
Flint, MI 48507
(313) 744-3600
Hotline: (800) 356-4357

National Council On Alcoholism
  & Addictions
202 East Boulevard Drive
Flint, MI 48503
(313) 767-0350

Grand Rapids

Care Unit Of Grand Rapids
1931 Boston Street SE
Grand Rapids, MI 49506
(616) 243-3608
Hotline: (800) 632-4556

Glenbeigh Of Kent
  Community Hospital
750 Fuller Avenue NE
Grand Rapids, MI 49503
(616) 242-6550
Hotline: (800) 422-0909

Occupational Health Centers
  Of America Inc.
400 Ann Street
Grand Rapids, MI 49506
(616) 363-4200
Hotline: (800) 523-0591

Holland

Family Services Of West Michigan
412 Century Lane
Holland, MI 49423
(616) 396-2301

Jackson

Bridgeway Center Inc.
301 Francis Street
Jackson, MI 49201
(517) 783-2732

Occupational Health Centers
  Of America
123 North West Avenue
Jackson, MI 49201
(517) 787-8933
Hotline: (800) 523-0591

Kalamazoo

Community Assessment &
  Screening
629 Pioneer Street
Kalamazoo, MI 49008
(616) 381-1510

Human Services Department
3299 Gull Road
Kalamazoo, MI 49001
(616) 373-5027
Hotline: (616) 381-4357

Lansing

National Council On Alcoholism
  & Drug Dependence
913 West Holmes Road
Lansing, MI 48910
(517) 394-1252
Hotline: (800) 344-3400

Total Health Education Inc.
3400 South Cedar Street
Lansing, MI 48911
(517) 393-5070

Livonia

Livonia Counseling Center
13325 Farmington Road
Livonia, MI 48150
(313) 261-3760

Marquette

Marquette General Hospital
Upper Michigan Rehabilitation
  Center
420 West Magnetic Street
Marquette, MI 49855
(906) 225-3160
Hotline: (906) 225-0155

Monroe

Monroe County Community
  Mental Health
1001 South Raisinville Road
Monroe, MI 48161
(313) 243-7340

Saginaw

Dot Caring Centers Inc.
3190 Hallmark Court
Saginaw, MI 48603
(517) 790-3366
Hotline: (800) 8CA-RING

Insight Recovery Center
420 North Michigan Avenue
Saginaw, MI 48602
(517) 754-2301
Hotline: (800) 356-HELP

Sault Sainte Marie

Marquette Medical Clinic
500 Osborne Boulevard
Sault Sainte Marie, MI 49783
(906) 632-0008

Southfield

Evergreen Counseling Centers
20755 Greenfield Road
Southfield, MI 48075
(313) 559-8790
Hotline: (800) 837-6424

Traverse City

Central Diagnostic &
  Referral Services
808A South Garfield Avenue
Traverse City, MI 49684
(616) 929-1315
Hotline: (800) 686-0749

Warren

Alcohol Evaluation Services
29200 Hoover Road
Warren, MI 48093
(313) 574-9644

MINNESOTA

Albert Lea

Fountain Lake Treatment Center
408 Fountain Street
Albert Lea, MN 56007
(507) 377-6411

Anoka

Riverplace Counseling Center
1806 South Ferry Street
Anoka, MN 55303
(612) 421-7924

Brainerd

Break Free
521 Charles Street
Brainerd, MN 56401
(218) 829-0307

Burnsville

Fairview Ridges
156 Cobblestone Lane
Burnsville, MN 55337
(612) 892-5962

Duluth

Center For Alcohol &
 Drug Treatment
314 West Superior Street
Duluth, MN 55802
(218) 722-4996

Minneapolis

Affirmation Place Ltd
127 West Grant Street
Minneapolis, MN 55403
(612) 871-9016

Lifestyle Counseling of Richfield
9801 DuPont Avenue South
Minneapolis, MN 55431
(612) 888-3511
Hotline: (612) 472-3444

Triumph Services
3735 Lakeland Avenue North
Minneapolis, MN 55422
(612) 522-5844

West Suburban Counseling Clinic
111 3rd Avenue South
Minneapolis, MN 55401
(612) 339-3787
Hotline: (612) 545-7907

Rochester

Guest House
4800 48th Street NE
Rochester, MN 55903
(507) 288-4693
Hotline: (800) 634-4155

Mayo Clinic
Baldwin Desk 3A
Rochester, MN 55905
(507) 284-4500

Saint Cloud

Saint Cloud Hospital
Recovery Plus
1406 North 6th Avenue
Saint Cloud, MN 56301
(612) 255-5612

Saint Paul

People Inc.
565 Dayton Avenue
Saint Paul, MN 55102
(612) 222-1009

Twin Town Treatment Center
1706 University Avenue
Saint Paul, MN 55104
(612) 645-3661

Thief River Falls

Glenmore Recovery Center
City Hall
Thief River Falls, MN 56701
(218) 681-7193
Hotline: (800) 584-9226

Winona

Hiawatha Valley Mental Hospital
111 Riverfront
Winona, MN 55987
(507) 454-4341

MISSISSIPPI

Columbus

Community Counseling Services
1001 Main Street
Columbus, MS 39701
(601) 328-9225
Hotline: (601) 323-4357

Gulfport

Gulf Coast Mental Health Center
4514 Old Pass Road
Gulfport, MS 39501
(601) 863-1132

Hattiesburg

Pine Grove Recovery Center
2255 Broadway Drive
Hattiesburg, MS 39401
(601) 264-0050
Hotline: (800) 821-7399

Jackson

Jackson Recovery Center
5354 I-55 South Frontage Road
Jackson, MS 39212
(601) 372-9788
Hotline: (800) 237-2122

National Council On Alcoholism
333 North Mart Plaza
Jackson, MS 39206
(601) 366-6880

Laurel

Serenity House
711 Royal Street
Laurel, MS 39440
(601) 428-7241

Meridian

Laurel Wood Center
5000 Highway 39 North
Meridian, MS 39305
(601) 483-6211
Hotline: (800) 422-5563

Pascagoula

Stevens Center
4905 Telephone Road
Pascagoula, MS 39567
(601) 769-1280
Hotline: (601) 769-1793

Vicksburg

Marian Hill Chemical
  Dependency Center
100 McCauley Drive
Vicksburg, MS 39180
(601) 631-2700
Hotline: (800) 843-2131

MISSOURI

Columbia

Comprehensive Human Service
409 Vandiver Drive
Columbia, MO 65202
(314) 874-8686

Farmington

SE Missouri Community
  Treatment Center
Highway 32 East
Farmington, MO 63640
(314) 756-5749
Hotline: (314) 756-6478

Fulton

Serve Inc.
1411 Airport Road
Fulton, MO 65251
(314) 642-0554

Hannibal

Hannibal Council On Alcohol
  & Drug Abuse Inc.
146 Communications Drive
Hannibal, MO 63401
(314) 248-1196

Kansas City

De La Salle Education Center
3740 Forest Avenue
Kansas City, MO 64109
(816) 561-4445
Hotline: (816) 435-0811

National Council On Alcoholism
  & Drug Dependence
601 East 63rd Street
Kansas City, MO 64110
(816) 361-5900

Research Mental Health Services
2801 Wyandotte Street
Kansas City, MO 64108
(816) 931-6500
Hotline: (816) 751-5151

Western Missouri Mental
  Health Center
600 East 22nd Street
Kansas City, MO 64108
(816) 471-300
Hotline: (816) 234-5980

Kennett

Family Counseling Center
925 Highway VV
Kennett, MO 63857
(314) 888-5925
Hotline: (314) 359-2600

Saint Joseph

Heartland Health System
801 Faraon Street
Heartland Hospital West
Saint Joseph, MO 64501
(816) 271-7312

Saint Louis

Cope & Twin Town Of Saint Louis
777 South New Ballas Street
Saint Louis, MO 63141
(314) 991-1819

Counseling Center Of Clayton
225 South Meramec Avenue
Saint Louis, MO 63105
(314) 725-6585

Deaconess Health Systems
530 Des Peres Road
Saint Louis, MO 63131
(314) 966-9248

Provident Counseling
9109 Watson Street
Saint Louis, MO 63126
(314) 533-8200
Hotline: (314) 469-9513

Springfield

Bridgeway Substance
  Abuse Program
2828 North National Avenue
Springfield, MO 65803
(417) 865-7575

Lakeland Regional Hospital
440 South Market Street
Springfield, MO 65806
(417) 865-5581
Hotline: (800) 432-1210

Ozarks National Council On
  Alcoholism & Drug Dependence
205 Saint Louis Street
Springfield, MO 65806
(417) 831-4167

MONTANA

Billings

Rimrock Foundation
1231 North 29th Street
Billings, MT 59101
(406) 248-3175
Hotline: (800) 227-3953

Deer Lodge

Chemical Dependency &
  Family Counseling Inc.
304 Milwaukee Avenue
Deer Lodge, MT 59722
(406) 846- 3442

Great Falls

Providence Center
401 3rd Avenue North
Great Falls, MT 59401
(406) 727-2512

Helena

Boyd Andrew Chemical
  Dependency Care Center
Arcade Building, Unit 1-E
Helena, MT 59601
(406) 443-2343

Kalispell

Glacier View Hospital
200 Heritage Way
Kalispell, MT 59901
(406) 752-5422
Hotline: (800) 843-2890

Miles City

Chemical Dependency Services Inc.
108 North Haynes Avenue
Miles City, MT 59301
(406) 232-6542

Missoula

Western Montana Regional
  Mental Health
500 North Higgins Street
Missoula, MT 59802
(406) 728-6817
Hotline: (406) 543-8623

Poplar

Spotted Bull Treatment Center
603 1/2 Court Avenue
Poplar, MT 59255
(406) 768-3852
Hotline: (800) 331-5298

NEBRASKA

Grand Island

Central Nebraska Council
  On Alcoholism
219 West 2nd Street
Grand Island, NE 68801
(308) 384-7365

Hastings

Council On Alcoholism & Drugs
432 North Minnesota Street
Hastings, NE 68901
(402) 463-0524

Lincoln

Alcoholism & Drug Abuse Council
650 J Street
Lincoln, NE 68508
(402) 474-0930
Hotline: (402) 648-4444

Lincoln Council Alcohol &
  Drugs Inc.
914 L Street
Lincoln, NE 68508
(402) 475-2694

Lincoln Lancaster Drug Projects Inc.
610 J Street
Lincoln, NE 68508
(402) 475-5161
Hotline: (402) 475-5683

Macy

Macy Youth & Family Services
Macy, NE 68039
(402) 837-5671

Norfolk

The Aware Program
103 North Street
Norfolk, NE 68701
(402) 370-3113
Hotline: (800) 672-8323

North Platte

Heartland Counseling &
  Consulting Clinic
110 North Bailey Street
North Platte, NE 69101
(308) 534-6029
Hotline: (308) 534-0440

Omaha

National Council On Alcoholism &
  Drug Dependence
115 North 49th Street
Omaha, NE 68132
(402) 553-8000

Operation Bridge Inc.
701 North 114th Street
Omaha, NE 68154
(402) 496-4777
Hotline: (800) 688-6082

Alcoholism Counseling Agency
2900 O Street
Omaha, NE 68107
(402) 734-3000

Scottsbluff

Panhandle Substance Abuse Council
1517 Broadway, Suite 124
Scottsbluff, NE 69361
(308) 632-3044

NEVADA

Carson City

Rural Clinics CMHC
Stewart Facility
Building 107
Carson City, NV 89710
(702) 687-5084
Hotline: (702) 323-6111

Elko

Ruby View Counseling Center
401 Railroad Street, Suite 301
Elko, NV 89801
(702) 738-8004
Hotline: (702) 738-0166

Las Vegas

Community Counseling Center
1006 East Sahara Avenue
Las Vegas, NV 89104
(702) 369-8700

Temporary Assistance For
 Domestic Crisis Shelter
Las Vegas, NV 89102
(702) 646-4981
Hotline: (702) 646-4981

Westcare Inc.
930 North 4th Street
Las Vegas, NV 89101
(702) 383-4044

Reno

Northern Area Substance
 Abuse Council
320 Flint Street
Reno, NV 89501
(702) 786-6563

Saint Marys Regional
 Medical Center
235 West 6th Street
Reno, NV 89520
(702) 789-3111

NEW HAMPSHIRE

Claremont

Counseling Center Of Claremont
241 Elm Street
Claremont, NH 03743
(603) 542-2578

Concord

Community Alcohol Information
 Program Inc.
10 Ferry Street
Concord, NH 03301
(603) 228-8181

Southeastern New Hampshire
 Services
105 Pleasant Street
Concord, NH 03301
(603) 225-9334
Hotline: (800) 698-7647

Dublin

Beech Hill Hospital
New Harrisville Road
Dublin, NH 03444
(603) 563-8511

Laconia

Horizons Counseling Center
390 Union Avenue
Laconia, NH 03246
(603) 524-8005

Manchester

National Council On Alcoholism
93-101 Manchester Street
Manchester, NH 03103
(603) 625-6980

Office Of Youth Services
66 Hanover Street
Manchester, NH 03101
(603) 624-6470

Nashua

Saint Josephs Hospital
172 Kinsley Street
Nashua, NH 03061
(603) 882-3000
Hotline: (800) 327-3331

NEW JERSEY

Bayonne

Community Mental Health Center
601 Broadway
Bayonne, NJ 07002
(201) 339-9200

Bridgeton

Cumberland County Alcoholism
& Drug Treatment
Cumberland County Medical Center
Cumberland Drive
Bridgeton, NJ 08302
(609) 455-8000

Camden

Alcove Drug & Alcohol
Treatment Program
1000 Atlantic Avenue
Camden, NJ 08104
(609) 342-4505

Cape May

Council On Alcoholism &
Drug Abuse Inc.
6 Moore Road
Cape May, NJ 08210
(609) 465-2282

Elizabeth

Elizabeth General Medical Center
655 East Jersey Street
Elizabeth, NJ 07201
(908) 965-7090

Flemington

National Council On Alcoholism &
Drug Dependence
153 Broad Street
Flemington, NJ 08822
(908) 782-3909

Hackensack

Alternatives To Domestic Violence
21 Main Street
Hackensack, NJ 07601
(201) 487-8484

Jersey City

Hudson County Council On
Alcoholism & Drug Abuse
83 Wayne Street
Jersey City, NJ 07302
(201) 451-2877
Hotline: (201) 451-2974

Lakewood

Alcoholism & Drug Abuse Council
Of Ocean County Inc.
117 East County Line Road
Lakewood, NJ 08701
(908) 367-5515

Morristown

Center For Addictive Illnesses
95 Mount Kemble Avenue
Morristown, NJ 07962
(201) 971-4700

New Brunswick

New Brunswick Counseling Center
84 New Street
New Brunswick, NJ 08903
(908) 246-4025

Newark

Integrity House Inc.
103 Lincoln Park
Newark, NJ 07102
(201) 623-0600
Hotline: (201) 623-5050

United Community Alcoholism
  Network
493 Clinton Avenue
Newark, NJ 07108
(201) 621-5663

Paramus

Bergen County Council On
  Alcoholism & Drugs Abuse Inc.
Bergen Pines Hospital Complex
Paramus, NJ 07652
(201) 261-2183

Paterson

Barnert Memorial Hospital Center
680 Broadway
Paterson, NJ 07514
(201) 977-6704

Plainfield

Plainfield Treatment Center
519 North Avenue
Plainfield, NJ 07060
(908) 757-8450

Somerville

Somerset Council On Alcoholism
  & Drug Dependency Inc.
112 Rehill Avenue
Somerville, NJ 08876
(908) 722-4900

Toms River

Ocean County Board Of
  Social Services
1027 Hooper Avenue
Toms River, NJ 08754
(908) 349-1500

Trenton

Helene Fuld Medical Center
750 Brunswick Avenue
Trenton, NJ 08638
(609) 394-6190
Hotline: (609) 394-6214

Mercer Council On Alcoholism &
  Drug Addiction
408 Bellevue Avenue
Trenton, NJ 08618
(609) 396-5874
Hotline: (800) 334-MEAS

NEW MEXICO

Albuquerque

Albuquerque Substance Abuse Clinic
117 Quincy Street NE
Albuquerque, NM 87108
(505) 260-1545

Charter Hospital Of Albuquerque
5901 Zuni Road SE
Albuquerque, NM 87108
(505) 265-8800
(800) 874-2476

Family Recovery Inc.
11805 Menaul Boulevard NE
Albuquerque, NM 87112
(505) 293-5146

Carlsbad

Carlsbad Mental Health Association
914 North Canal Street
Carlsbad, NM 88220
(505) 885-4836
Hotline: (505) 885-8888

Farmington

Meyers Counseling Services
2124 North Sullivan Avenue
Farmington, NM 87401
(505) 327-2066
Hotline: (505) 325-0398

Gallup

Behavioral Health Services
650 Van den Bosch Parkway
Gallup, NM 87301
(505) 722-3804
Hotline: (800) 722-3804

Las Cruces

Southwest Counseling Center Inc.
1480 North Main Street
Las Cruces, NM 88005
(505) 526-3371

Sante Fe

Pinon Hills Hospital
313 Camino Alire
Sante Fe, NM 87501
(800) 234-8000

NEW YORK

Albany

Aids Council Of Northeastern
  New York
Alcoholism Prevention Education
750 Broadway
Albany, NY 12207
(518) 434-4686

Al Care
445 New Karner Road
Albany, NY 12205
(518) 456-8043

Albany Citizens Council On
  Alcoholism & Other Chemical
  Dependencies Inc.
283 Central Avenue
Albany, NY 12206
(518) 465-5829

Colonie Youth Center
1653 Central Avenue
Albany, NY 12205
(518) 869-8328

Saint Peters Addiction
  Recovery Center
315 South Manning Boulevard
Albany, NY 12208
(518) 454-1307

Batavia

Genesee Council On Alcoholism
  & Substance Abuse Inc.
30 Bank Street
Batavia, NY 14020
(716) 343-1124
Hotline: (716) 343-1124

Binghamton

Broome County Council
  On Alcoholism
25 Main Street
Binghamton, NY 13905
(607) 723-7529

United Health Services
24-42 Mitchell Avenue
Binghamton, NY 13903
(607) 762-3232
Hotline: (800) 445-3569

Bronx

Bronx Committee For The
  Betterment Of Alcoholism
  Services In The Bronx
3164 3rd Avenue
Bronx, NY 10451
(718) 402-8900

Our Lady Of Mercy Medical Center
Alcoholism Outpatient Clinic
4401 Bronx Boulevard
Bronx, NY 10470
(718) 920-9100

Seneca Center Inc.
1241 Lafayette Avenue
Bronx, NY 10474
(718) 542-6130

South Fordham Organization Inc.
2385 Valentine Avenue
Bronx, NY 10458
(718) 295-4130

Brooklyn

Brooklyn Addiction Task Force Inc.
465 Dean Street
Brooklyn, NY 11217
(718) 783-0883

Coney Island Hospital
2601 Ocean Parkway
Brooklyn, NY 11235
(718) 615-5972

Cumberland Diagnostic &
   Treatment Center
100 North Portland Avenue
Brooklyn, NY 11205
(718) 403-0869

Kings County Hospital Center
606 Winthrop Street
Brooklyn, NY 11203
(718) 735-2723

Lutheran Medical Center
514 49th Street
Brooklyn, NY 11220
(718) 854-2041

Buffalo

Erie County Medical Center
462 Grider Street
Buffalo, NY 14215
(716) 898-3415
Hotline: (716) 898-3471

Greater Buffalo Council On
   Alcoholism & Substance Abuse
220 Delaware Avenue
Buffalo, NY 14202
(716) 852-1781

Mid Erie Alcoholism
   Outpatient Clinic
463 William Street
Buffalo, NY 14204
(716) 852-0383
Hotline: (716) 834-3131

Elmira

Alcohol & Drug Abuse Council
   Of Chemung County
380 West Gray Street
Elmira, NY 14905
(607) 734-1567

Flushing

Long Island Consultation Center Inc.
97-29 64th Road
Flushing, NY 11374
(718) 896-3400

Freeport

South Shore Child
   Guidance Center
Care Alcoholism Program
87 Church Street
Freeport, NY 11520
(516) 378-2992

Happauge

Suffolk County Alcoholism
   Community Education &
   Intervention
900 Wheeler Road
Happauge, NY 11788
(516) 366-1717

Hempstead

Family Services Association Of
  Nassau County
126 North Franklin Avenue
Hempstead, NY 11550
(516) 486-7200

Huntington Station

Long Island Association For
  Aids Care Inc.
1335 New York Avenue
Huntington Station, NY 11746
(516) 385-2451

Ithaca

Alcoholism Council Of
  Tompkins County
201 East Green Street
Ithaca, NY 14850
(607) 274-6288

Jamaica

Outreach Development Corporation
89-15 Woodhaven Boulevard
Jamaica, NY 11421
(718) 847-9233

Queens Hospital Center
82-68 164th Street
Jamaica, NY 11432
(718) 883-2750

Kingston

Alcohol & Substance
  Abuse Council
785 Broadway
Kingston, NY 12401
(914) 331-9331

Manhasset

The Long Island Home Ltd.
535 Plandome Road
Manhasset, NY 11030
(516) 365-8806
Hotline: (800) 732-9808

Middletown

Middletown Community
  Health Center
14 Grove Street
Middletown, NY 10940
(914) 343-8838

Monticello

Sullivan County MH/MR
  Alcoholism Services
17 Hamilton Avenue
Monticello, NY 12701
(914) 794-0761

New Rochellle

United Hospital
3 The Boulevard
New Rochelle, NY 10801
(914) 235-6633

New York

Alcoholism Council Of
  Greater New York
49 East 21st Street
New York, NY 10010
(212) 979-6277

BRC Human Services Corporation
324 Lafayette Street
New York, NY 10012
(212) 925-9393

Central Harlem Emergency
  Care Services
419 West 126th Street
New York, NY 10027
(212) 865-6133

Enter Inc.
302-306 East 111th Street
New York, NY 10029
(212) 876-2525

Greenwich House Inc.
55 5th Avenue
New York, NY 10003
(212) 463-8244

Inter Care Inc.
51 East 25th Street
New York, NY 10010
(212) 532-0303

Inwood Community Services Inc.
651 Academy Street
New York, NY 10034
(212) 942-0043

Manhattan Alcoholism
  Treatment Center
600 East 125th Street
Wards Island
New York, NY 10035
(212) 369-0322

NY Center For Addiction Treatment
568 Broadway
New York, NY 10012
(212) 966-9537

Newburgh

City Of Newburgh Youth Bureau
167 Broadway
Newburgh, NY 12550
(914) 565-1213

Niagara Falls

Alcohol Council In Niagara County
800 Main Street
Niagara Falls, NY 14301
(716) 282-1228

Nyack

Rockland Council On Alcoholism Inc.
11 Division Avenue
Nyack, NY 10960
(914) 358-4357

Plainview

Nassau County Department Of
  Drug & Alcohol
1425 Old Country Road
Plainview, NY 11803
(516) 420-5033

Poughkeepsie

Dutchess County Council On
  Alcoholism & Chemical
  Dependency Inc.
20 Maple Street
Poughkeepsie, NY 12601
(914) 471-0194

Riverhead

Riverhead Community Awareness
  Program Inc.
542 East Main Street
Riverhead, NY 11901
(516) 727-3722

Rochester

Family Services Of Rochester Inc.
30 Clinton Avenue North
Rochester, NY 14604
(716) 232-1840

Monroe County Office Of
  Mental Health
375 Westfall Road
Rochester, NY 14620
(716) 274-6144

Schenectady

Alcoholism Council Of
  Schenectady County Inc.
302 State Street
Schenectady, NY 12305
(518) 346-4457

Staten Island

Staten Island MH Society Inc.
30 Nelson Avenue
Staten Island, NY 10308
(718) 966-1296

Staten Island University Hospital
475 Seaview Avenue
Staten Island, NY 10305
(718) 226-2752
Hotline: (718) 226-2791

Syracuse

Child & Family Service Of
 Onondaga County
450 South Main Street
Syracuse, NY 13212
(315) 458-8100

Onandaga Council On
 Alcoholism Inc.
716 James Street
Syracuse, NY 13203
(315) 471-1359
Hotline: (315) 472-3784

Troy

Rensselaer County MH
 Unified Services
7th Avenue
County Office Building
Troy, NY 12180
(518) 270-2800

Utica

Oneida County Department
 Of Mental Health
800 Park Avenue
Utica, NY 13501
(315) 798-5676

White Plains

National Council On Alcoholism
360 Mamaroneck Avenue
White Plains, NY 10605
(914) 683-1213

NORTH CAROLINA

Asheville

Woodhill Treatment Center
60 Caledonia Road
Asheville, NC 28803
(704) 253-3681

Charlotte

Charlotte Council On Alcoholism
 & Chemical Dependency Inc.
100 Billingsley Road
Charlotte, NC 28211
(704) 376-7447

Mecklenburg County Area
 MH Authority
429 Billingsley Road
Charlotte, NC 28211
(704) 336-2023

Durham

Durham Council On Alcoholism &
 Drug Dependency Inc.
3109 University Drive
Durham, NC 27707
(919) 493-3114

Greensboro

Guilford County Mental
 Health Center
201 North Eugene Street
Greensboro, NC 27401
(919) 373-3630

Substance Abuse Services
 Of Guilford
1305 Glenwood Avenue
Greensboro, NC 27403
(919) 373-3080

Morganton

Foothills Area Mental
 Health Center
1001 B East Union Street
Morganton, NC 28655
(704) 438-6226
Hotline: (800) 942-1797

Raleigh

Drug Action Inc.
2809 Industrial Drive
Raleigh, NC 27609
(919) 832-4453

Salisbury

Rowan Memorial Hospital
612 Mocksville Avenue
Salisbury, NC 28144
(704) 638-1300

Winston-Salem

Charter Hospital Of
  Winston-Salem
3637 Old Vineyard Road
Winston-Salem, NC 27104
(919) 768-7710
Hotline: (800) 441-2673

NORTH DAKOTA

Bismarck

Burleigh County Detoxification
  Center
514 East Thayer Avenue
Bismarck, ND 58501
(701) 222-6651
Hotline: (701) 222-6656

Fargo

Professional Resource Network
1323 23rd Street South
Fargo, ND 58103
(701) 235-2735

Southeast Human Service Center
2624 9th Avenue South
Fargo, ND 58103
(701) 298-4500
Hotline: (701) 235-7335

Grand Forks

Northeast Human Service Center
1407 24th Avenue South
Grand Forks, ND 58201
(701) 746-9411
Hotline: (701) 775-0525

Jamestown

South Central Human Service Center
520 3rd Street NW
Jamestown, ND 58402
(701) 252-2641

Minot

North Central Human Service Center
400 22nd Avenue NW
Minot, ND 58701
(701) 852-1251

OHIO

Akron

Akron Health Department
177 South Broadway
Akron, OH 44308
(216) 375-2984

Family Services
3050 West Market Street
Akron, OH 44333
(216) 873-4720

Canton

Quest Recovery Services Inc.
1341 Market Avenue North
Canton, OH 44714
(216) 453-8252

Cincinnati

Alcoholism Council Of
  Cincinnati Area
118 William Howard Taft Road
Cincinnati, OH 45219
(513) 281-7880
Hotline: (513) 721-7900

Talbert House
100 Shadybrook Drive
Cincinnati, OH 45216
(513) 761-9117

Cleveland

Alcohol & Drug Recovery Center
9500 Euclid Avenue
Cleveland, OH 44195
(216) 444-8739

Alcoholism Services Of Cleveland
14805 Detroit Avenue
Cleveland, OH 44118
(216) 226-2844

Metro Health Clement Center
2500 East 79th Street
Cleveland, OH 44104
(216) 391-3200
Hotline: (216) 371-5656

Columbus

Intervention & Assessment
  Program
1375 South Hamilton Road
Columbus, OH 43227
(614) 235-2070

North Central Mental
  Health Services
1301 North High Street
Columbus, OH 43201
(614) 299-6600
Hotline: (614) 221-5445

Parkside Lodge
349 Ridenour Road
Columbus, OH 43230
(614) 471-2552
Hotline: (800) 727-5743

Dayton

Combined Health District Center
  For Alcohol & Drug Addiction
  Services
4100 West 3rd Street
Dayton, OH 45428
(513) 268-0141

South Community Inc.
8353 Yankee Street
Dayton, OH 45458
(513) 435-6660

Hamilton

Drug Counseling Services Of
  Butler County Inc.
202 South Monument Street
Hamilton, OH 45011
(513) 863-1100

Lima

Northwest Center For Human
  Resources
529 South Elizabeth Street
Lima, OH 45804
(419) 228-5508
Hotline: (800) 445-3333

Mansfield

Center For Individual &
  Family Services
741 Scholl Street
Mansfield, OH 44907
(419) 756-1717
Hotline: (419) 522-4357

Newark

Licking County Alcoholism
  Prevention Program
62 East Steven Street
Newark, OH 43055
(614) 366-7303

Sandusky

Alcohol Education &
  Assessment Program
209 East Water Street
Sandusky, OH 44870
(419) 626-5398

Springfield

McKinley Hall Inc.
1101 East High Street
Springfield, OH 45505
(513) 328-5300

Toledo

Comprehensive Addiction
  Service Systems
2465 Collingwood Boulevard
Toledo, OH 43620
(419) 241-8827
Hotline: (419) 241-1014

Warren

Addiction Recovery Center Of
  Hillside Hospital
8747 Squires Lane NE
Warren, OH 44484
(216) 841-3805
Hotline: (216) 841-3859

Youngstown

Alcoholic Clinic Of Youngstown
2151 Rush Boulevard
Youngstown, OH 44507
(216) 744-1181
Hotline: (800) 228-8287

OKLAHOMA

Ardmore

MH Services Of Southern
  Oklahoma
2530 South Commerce Street
Ardmore, OK 73401
(405) 223-5070
Hotline: (800) 522-1090

Lawton

Area Prevention Resource Center
116 NW 31st Street
Lawton, OK 73505
(405) 355-5246

Miami

Northeastern Oklahoma Council
  On Alcoholism
316 Eastgate Boulevard
Miami, OK 74355
(918) 542-2845

Oklahoma City

Community Counseling Center
1140 North Hudson Street
Oklahoma City, OK 73103
(405) 272-0660

The Referral Center For Alcoholism
  & Drug Service Of Central
  Oklahoma Inc.
1215 NW 25th Street
Oklahoma City, OK 73106
(405) 525-2525

Tulsa

Associated Centers For Therapy Inc.
7010 South Yale Street
Tulsa, OK 74136
(918) 492-2554
Hotline: (800) 722-3611

Health Network Inc.
2326 South Garnett Street
Tulsa, OK 74129
(918) 664-2907
Hotline: (800) 468-5901

Tulsa Area Council On Alcoholism
  & Drug Abuse
4828 South Peoria Street
Tulsa, OK 74105
(918) 495-3883
Hotline: (918) 742-5600

OREGON

Eugene

Addiction Counseling &
  Education Services Inc.
1639 Oak Street
Eugene, OR 97401
(503) 344-2237

Buckley House Programs Inc.
605 West 4th Street
Eugene, OR 97402
(503) 343-6512
Hotline: (503) 343-3550

Portland

CODA Drug Treatment Services
306 NE 20th Street
Portland, OR 97232
(503) 239-8400

Counseling Intervention
 Programs Inc.
4413 SE 17th Street
Portland, OR 97202
(503) 230-9654

Project For Community Recovery
3525 NE Martin Luther King Jr
 Boulevard
Portland, OR 97212
(503) 281-2804

Roseburg

Douglas County Council On
 Alcohol & Drug Abuse
Prevention & Treatment
621 West Madrone Street
Roseburg, OR 97470
(503) 672-2691
Hotline: (503) 672-2692

Salem

Marion County Drug Treatment
 Program
3180 Center Street NE
Salem, OR 97301
(503) 588-5358

Serenity Lane
755 Medical Center Drive NE
Salem, OR 97301
(503) 588-2804
Hotline: (503) 687-1110

PENNSYLVANIA

Allentown

Council On Alcohol & Drug Abuse
126 North 9th Street
Allentown, PA 18102
(215) 437-0801

Altoona

Blair County Community
 Action Program
5433 Industrial Avenue
Altoona, PA 16601
(814) 946-3651

Butler

Butler County Council On
 Alcoholism & Drug Dependency
227 South Chestnut Street
Butler, PA 16001
(412) 287-5294
Hotline: (412) 776-1113

Chester

Crozer Chester Medical Center
1 East 9th Street
Chester, PA 19013
(215) 499-5440
Hotline: (215) 447-6081

Doylestown

Bucks County Council On
 Alcoholism & Drug Dependence
252 West Swamp Road
Doylestown, PA 18901
(215) 345-6644
Hotline: (800) 221-6333

Erie

GECAC Drug & Alcohol Services
809 Peach Street
Erie, PA 16501
(814) 459-4581
Hotline: (814) 870-5424

Harrisburg

Greater Harrisburg Alcohol &
 Drug Counseling
3309 Spring Street
Harrisburg, PA 17109
(717) 545-5011

Lancaster

Lancaster Clinical Counseling
 Association
131 East Orange Street
Lancaster, PA 17602
(717) 299-0131

Media

Alcoholism & Addictions Council
 Of Delaware County
115 West State Street
Media, PA 19063
(215) 566-8143
Hotline: (215) 566-8144

Philadelphia

Bridge Counseling Center
1912 Welsh Road
Philadelphia, PA 19115
(215) 969-8990

Intercommunity Action Inc.
6122 Ridge Avenue
Philadelphia, PA 19128
(215) 487-1981
Hotline: (215) 483-8255

Jefferson Outreach Drug &
 Alcohol Program
1201 Chestnut Street
Philadelphia, PA 19107
(215) 955-8856

The Assistance Program
1225 Vine Street
Philadelphia, PA 19107
(215) 665-1730

Pittsburgh

Abraxas Foundation Inc.
936 West North Street
Pittsburgh, PA 15233
(412) 323-9221
Hotline: (800) ABR-AXAS

Saint Francis Medical Center
400 45th Street
Pittsburgh, PA 15201
(412) 622-7622
Hotline: (412) 622-4631

Reading

Center For Mental Health
6th & Spruce Streets
Reading, PA 19611
(215) 378-6186

Wilkes-Barre

Luzerne/Wyoming Counties
111 North Pennsylvania Boulevard
Wilkes-Barre, PA 18701
(717) 826-8790
Hotline: (717) 829-1341

RHODE ISLAND

Cranston

Alcoholism Services Of Cranston/
 Johnson & NW Rhode Island
311 Doric Avenue
Cranston, RI 02910
(401) 781-3990

Newport

Community Organization For
 Drug Abuse Control
93 Thames Street
Newport, RI 02840
(401) 846-4150

Pawtucket

Rhode Island Council On
  Alcoholism
500 Prospect Street
Pawtucket, RI 02860
(401) 725-0410
Hotline: (800) 622-7422

Providence

Providence Center For Counseling
  & Psychiatric Services
790 North Main Street
Providence, RI 02904
(401) 861-6262

Talbot Treatment Centers Inc.
265 Oxford Street
Providence, RI 02905
(401) 785-8383
Hotline: (401) 785-8384

Warwick

Counseling & Intervention
  Services Inc.
3649 Post Road
Warwick, RI 02886
(401) 738-1240

Woonsocket

Northern RI Community MH
  Center Inc.
181 Cumberland Street
Woonsocket, RI 02895
(401) 766-3330
Hotline: (401) 762-1577

SOUTH CAROLINA

Anderson

Anderson/Oconee Counties Alcohol
  & Drug Abuse Commission
212 South Main Street
Anderson, SC 29624
(803) 260-4168
Hotline: (803) 225-0297

Charleston

Charleston County Substance
  Abuse Commission
25 Courtenay Drive
Charleston, SC 29401
(803) 723-7212

Columbia

Lexington/Richland Alcohol &
  Drug Abuse Council
1325 Harden Street
Columbia, SC 29204
(803) 256-3100

Conway

Coastal Carolina Hospital
152 Waccamaw Medical Park Drive
Conway, SC 29526
(803) 347-7156
Hotline: (800) 922-0742

Lancaster

Lancaster County Commission On
  Alcohol & Drug Abuse
114 South Main Street
Lancaster, SC 29720
(803) 285-6912

Spartanburg

Spartanburg County Commission
  On Alcohol & Drug Abuse
131 North Spring Street
Spartanburg, SC 29306
(803) 582-7588
Hotline: (803) 591-4425

Winnsboro

Fairfield County Substance Abuse
  Commission
200 Calhoun Street
Winnsboro, SC 29180
(803) 635-2335

SOUTH DAKOTA

Aberdeen

Northern Alcohol/Drug Referral &
 Information Center
221 South First Street
Aberdeen, SD 57402
(605) 225-6131
Hotline: (605) 229-7640

Huron

Our Home Inc,
510 Nebraska Avenue SW
Huron, SD 57350
(605) 353-1025
Hotline: (800) 351-1477

Rapid City

City/County Receiving & Referral
 Center
725 North Lacrosse Street
Rapid City, SD 57701
(605) 394-6128

Sioux Falls

Carroll Institutes
231 South Phillips Avenue
Sioux Falls, SD 57102
(605) 332-5542

First Step Counseling Services
5201 West 41st Street
Sioux Falls, SD 57106
(605) 361-1505

Watertown

Human Service Agency
123 19th Street NE
Watertown, SD 57201
(605) 886-7602
Hotline: (605) 886-5841

Yankton

Lewis & Clark Mental
 Health Center
1028 Walnut Street
Yankton, SD 57058
(605) 665-6508
Hotline: (605) 665-4606

TENNESSEE

Chattanooga

Council For Alcohol & Drug
 Abuse Services
207 Spears Avenue
Chattanooga, TN 37405
(615) 756-7644
Hotline: (615) 756-7645

Jackson

Jackson Area Council On
 Alcoholism & Drug Dependency
900 East Chester Street
Jackson, TN 38301
(901) 423-3653

Johnson City

Comprehensive Community
 Services
323 West Walnut Street
Johnson City, TN 37604
(615) 928-6581
Hotline: (800) 628-0075

Knoxville

Knoxville Community Action
 Committee
2247 Western Avenue
Knoxville, TN 37921
(615) 522-5197

Memphis

Memphis Alcohol & Drug Council
1450 Poplar Street
Memphis, TN 38104
(901) 274-0056

Northeast Community Mental
 Health Center
5515 Shelby Oaks Drive
Memphis, TN 38134
(901) 382-3880
Hotline: (901) 577-9400

Southeast Mental Health Center Inc.
3810 Winchester Road
Memphis, TN 38118
(901) 369-1400

Nashville

Alcohol & Drug Council Of Middle
 Tennessee Inc.
2612 Westwood Drive
Nashville, TN 37204
(615) 269-0029

MCC Managed Behavioral Care Inc.
2416 21st Avenue South
Nashville, TN 37212
(615) 383-5082

Oak Ridge

Hope Of East Tennessee Inc.
176 Northwestern Avenue
Oak Ridge, TN 37830
(615) 482-4826

TEXAS

Abilene

Hendrick Medical Center
190 Woodlawn Drive
Abilene, TX 79603
(915) 670-5050

Austin

Austin Drug & Alcohol Abuse
 Program
13377 Pond Springs Road
Austin, TX 78729
(512) 219-8180

Austin Travis County MH/MR Oak
 Springs Treatment Center
3000 Oak Springs Drive
Austin, TX 78702
(512) 926-5301
Hotline: (512) 472-4357

Greater Austin Council On
 Alcoholism & Drug Abuse Inc.
1609 Shoal Creek Street
Austin, TX 78701
(512) 873-8191
Hotline: (800) 533-0714

Beaumont

Charter Counseling Center
 Of Beaumont
85 IH-10 North
Beaumont, TX 77707
(409) 839-4882
Hotline: (800) 256-1552

Bryan

MH/MR Authority Of Brazos Valley
623 Mary Lake Drive
Bryan, TX 77801
(409) 846-6935
Hotline: (800) 282-6467

Corpus Christi

Nueces County MH/MR Center
1546 South Brownlee Street
Corpus Christi, TX 78404
(512) 886-6970
Hotline: (512) 886-6965

Dallas

Charlton Methodist Hospital
3500 Wheatland Road
Dallas, TX 75237
(214) 709-9800
Hotline: (214) 709-9800

First Step Counseling Center
13612 Midway Road
Dallas, TX 75244
(214) 239-4440

Metropolitan Clinic Of
  Counseling Inc.
12720 Hillcrest Road
Dallas, TX 75230
(214) 701-0482
Hotline: (800) 283-6226

El Paso

Genesis Recovery Center
6070 Gateway East
El Paso, TX 79905
(915) 775-1976
Hotline: (800) 460-1976

Life Management Center For MH/
  MR Services
1014 North Stanton Street
El Paso, TX 79901
(915) 542-4971
Hotline: (915) 779-1800

Fort Worth

Family Service Inc.
1424 Hemphill Street
Fort Worth, TX 76104
(817) 927-5544

Tarrant Council On Alcoholism &
  Drug Abuse
1200 Summit Avenue
Fort Worth, TX 76102
(817) 332-6329

Greenville

Crossroads Council On Alcohol &
  Drug Abuse
2612 Jordan Street
Greenville, TX 75401
(214) 455-5438
Hotline: (800) 397-5448

Harlingen

South Texas Hospital
1/2 Mile South Rangerville Road
Harlingen, TX 78550
(512) 423-3420 ext. 444

Houston

Gulf Coast Community Services
  Association
6300 Bowling Green Street
Houston, TX 77021
(713) 748-4410

Houston Council On Alcohol &
  Drug Abuse
4605 Wilmington Street
Houston, TX 77051
(713) 520-5502

Metropolitan Clinic Of
  Counseling Inc.
1900 West Loop South
Houston, TX 77027
(800) 933-8816

Volunteers Of America
312 East Rogers Street
Houston, TX 77022
(713) 692-8190

Lubbock

Lubbock Regional MH/MR Center
1202 Main Street
Lubbock, TX 79401
(806) 766-0251

Lufkin

Alcohol & Drug Abuse Council Of
  Deep East Texas
304 North Raguet Street
Lufkin, TX 75901
(409) 634-5753
Hotline: (800) 445-8562

Midland

Permian Basin Community Centers
  For MH/MR
3701 North Big Spring Street
Midland, TX 79701
(915) 570-3385
Hotline: (915) 570-5300

Plainview

Central Plains Center For
 MH/MR/SA
620 West 7th Street
Plainview, TX 79072
(806) 293-0190
Hotline: (806) 296-5555

San Angelo

San Angelo Council On Alcohol &
 Drug Abuse
1021 Caddo Street
San Angelo, TX 76901
(915) 655-9641
Hotline: (800) 880-9641

San Antonio

Alamo Mental Health Group Inc.
4242 Medical Drive
San Antonio, TX 78229
(210) 616-0074

South Texas Counseling Centers Inc.
11330 IH 10 West
San Antonio, TX 78249
(512) 736-1911

Temple

Central Counties Center For
 MH/MR Services
304 South 22nd Street
Temple, TX 76501
(817) 778-4841
Hotline: (817) 526-4146

Texarkana

Choices
301 Westlawn Drive
Texarkana, TX 75501
(903) 832-1489

Waco

Providence Health Center
6901 Medical Parkway
Waco, TX 76712
(817) 751-4000
Hotline: (817) 776-5970

Wichita Falls

Helen Farabee Center
500 South Broad Street
Wichita Falls, TX 76301
(817) 322-1585
Hotline: (817) 322-1196

UTAH

Ogden

McKay/Dee Hospital
5030 Harrison Boulevard
Ogden, UT 84403
(801) 476-5777
Hotline: (801) 476-5600

Orem

Utah County Council On Drug
 Abuse Rehabilitation
555 South State Street
Orem, UT 84058
(801) 226-2255

Provo

Utah County Division Of
 Substance Abuse
100 East Center
Provo, UT 84606
(801) 370-8427

Salt Lake City

Salt Lake County Alcohol
 Counseling & Education Center
231 East 400 South
Salt Lake City, UT 84111
(801) 538-2279

University Of Utah
Alcohol & Drug Abuse Clinic
50 North Medical Drive
Salt Lake City, UT 84132
(801) 581-6228

Utah Alcoholism Foundation
2880 South Main Street
Salt Lake City, UT 84115
(801) 487-3276
Hotline: (800) 345-4828

VERMONT

Brattleboro

Youth Services Inc.
11 Walnut Street
Brattleboro, VT 05301
(802) 257-0361

Burlington

Howard Mental Health Services
300 Flynn Avenue
Burlington, VT 05401
(802) 658-0404
Hotline: (802) 656-3587

Middlebury

Counseling Service Of Addison
  County
89 Main Street
Middlebury, VT 05753
(802) 388-6751

Saint Johnsbury

Northeastern Vermont Regional
  Hospital
Hospital Drive
Saint Johnsbury, VT 05819
(802) 748-8141
Hotline: (800) 243-7262

Springfield

Canterbury Counseling Services
374 North River Road
Springfield, VT 05156
(802) 886-2577
Hotline: (800) 639-8036

Waterbury

VT Office Of Alcohol & Drug
  Abuse Programs
102 South Main Street
Waterbury, VT 05671
(802) 241-2170

VIRGINIA

Alexandria

Alexandria Community
  Services Board
2344-A Mill Road
Alexandria, VA 22314
(703) 329-2020

Arlington

Arlington Alcohol Safety
  Action Program
1400 North Courthouse Road
Arlington, VA 22201
(703) 358-4420

Danville

Danville/Pittsylvania MH
  Services Board
245 Hairston Street
Danville, VA 24540
(804) 799-0456
Hotline: (804) 793-4922

Hampton

Peninsula Hospital
Adult Chemical Dependency Unit
2244 Executive Drive
Hampton, VA 23666
(804) 827-1001
Hotline: (800) 759-1001

Newport News

Peninsula Alcoholism Services
732 Thimble Shoals Boulevard
Newport News, VA 23606
(804) 594-7321

Portsmouth

Portsmouth Community
  Services Board
500 Crawford Street
Portsmouth, VA 23704
(804) 393-8618

Richmond

Human Resources Inc.
2926 West Marshall Street
Richmond, VA 23230
(804) 355-8478
Hotline: (804) 355-2176

Winchester

New Life Counseling Services
19 North Washington Street
Winchester, VA 22601
(703) 722-6187
Hotline: (800) 545-5433

WASHINGTON

Bellevue

Eastside Alcohol/Drug Center
606 120th Avenue NE
Bellevue, WA 98005
(206) 454-1505

Bellingham

Unitycare
202 Unity Street
Bellingham, WA 98225
(206) 647-2341
Hotline: (800) 640-2599

Everett

Community Alcohol &
  Drug Services
2808 Hoyt Avenue
Everett, WA 98201
(206) 258-2662

Olympia

Community Mental Health Center
112 East State Street
Olympia, WA 98501
(206) 943-7177

Seattle

Alcohol/Drug 24 Hour Help Line
5700 Rainier Avenue South
Seattle, WA 98144
(206) 722-3703
Hotline: (800) 562-1240

Central Seattle Recovery Center
1401 East Jefferson Street
Seattle, WA 98122
(206) 322-2970

South King County Drug &
  Alcohol Recovery Centers
15025 4th Avenue SW
Seattle, WA 98166
(206) 242-3506

Spokane

Addiction Outpatient Services
11704 East Montgomery Drive
Spokane, WA 99206
(509) 928-6963

Colonial Clinic
West 315 9th Avenue
Spokane, WA 99204
(509) 838-6004
Hotline: (509) 466-2772

Mountainview Outpatient
517 South Division Street
Spokane, WA 99202
(509) 456-0831
Hotline: (800) 926-0048

Tacoma

Pierce County Alliance
1110 South 12th Avenue
Tacoma, WA 98405
(206) 591-6090

Western Washington Alcohol
Center Inc.
3049 South 36th Street
Tacoma, WA 98409
(206) 536-5549

Vancouver

Clark County Council On
Alcohol & Drugs
509 West 8th Street
Vancouver, WA 98660
(206) 696-1631

Yakima

A J Alcohol & Drug Services
32 North 3rd Street
Yakima, WA 98901
(509) 248-0133
Hotline: (800) 922-2015

WEST VIRGINIA

Beckley

Fayette/Monroe/Raleigh/Summers
Mental Health Council Inc.
101 South Eisenhower Drive
Beckley, WV 25801
(304) 256-7100

Charleston

Charleston Area Medical Center Inc.
Brooks & Washington Streets
Charleston, WV 25325
(304) 348-6060

Huntington

HCA River Park Hospital
1230 6th Avenue
Huntington, WV 25701
(304) 526-9111
Hotline: (800) 621-2673

Morgantown

Chestnut Ridge Hospital
930 Chestnut Ridge Road
Morgantown, WV 26505
(304) 293-4000
Hotline: (800) 458-4898

Wheeling

Northwood Health Systems
2121 Eoff Street
Wheeling, WV 26003
(304) 234-3570

WISCONSIN

Appleton

Saint Elizabeth Hospital
1506 South Oneida Street
Appleton, WI 54915
(414) 738-2389
Hotline: (800) 223-7332

Beloit

Addiction Treatment &
Education Program
2091 Shopiere Road
Beloit, WI 53511
(608) 364-1144

Chippewa Falls

Council On Alcohol & Other
Drug Abuse
404 1/2 North Bridge Street
Chippewa Falls, WI 54729
(715) 723-1101
Hotline: (800) 428-8159

Eau Claire

Midelfort Clinic
733 West Clairemont Avenue
Eau Claire, WI 54701
(715) 839-5369

Green Bay

Brown County Mental Health Center
2900 Saint Anthony Drive
Green Bay, WI 54311
(414) 468-1136

Janesville

Rock County Psychiatric Hospital
Substance Abuse Services
3530 North City Trunk F
Janesville, WI 53545
(608) 757-4848
Hotline: (608) 757-5025

Kenosha

Alcohol & Other Drugs Council
 Of Kenosha County Inc.
1115 56th Street
Kenosha, WI 53140
(414) 658-8166

La Crosse

Coulee Council On Alcohol &
 Other Chemical Abuse
921 West Avenue South
La Crosse, WI 54601
(608) 784-4177

Madison

Madison Inner City Council On
 Substance Abuse Inc.
1244 South Park Street
Madison, WI 53715
(608) 257-4066

Prevention & Intervention Center
 For Alcohol & Other Drug Abuse
2000 Fordem Avenue
Madison, WI 53704
(608) 246-7600

Milwaukee

Inner City Council On Alcoholism
3660 North Teutonia Avenue
Milwaukee, WI 53206
(414) 871-5181

Milwaukee Council On Alcoholism
2266 North Prospect Avenue
Milwaukee, WI 53202
(414) 276-8487
Hotline: (414) 271-3123

Psychological Addiction Consultants
5401 North 76th Street
Milwaukee, WI 53218
(414) 535-0072

Oshkosh

Winnebago County Department
 Of Community Programs
471 High Avenue
Oshkosh, WI 54901
(414) 236-4734
Hotline: (414) 233-7707

Racine

Crisis Center Of Racine Inc.
209 8th Street
Racine, WI 53403
(414) 637-9898

Sheboygan

Counseling & Development Center
2205 Erie Avenue
Sheboygan, WI 53081
(414) 459-8871

Stevens Point

Community Alcohol & Drug
 Abuse Center
209 Prentice Street North
Stevens Point, WI 54481
(715) 344-4611
Hotline: (715) 345-0711

Waukesha

Waukesha County Council On
 Alcoholism & Drug Abuse
310 South Street
Waukesha, WI 53186
(414) 524-7921
Hotline: (414) 524-7920

WYOMING

Casper

Central Wyoming Counseling
  Center
1200 East 3rd Street
Casper, WY 82601
(307) 237-9583

Cheyenne

Southeast Wyoming Mental
  Health Center
1609 East 19th Street
Cheyenne, WY 82001
(307) 632-9361
Hotline: (307) 632-6433

Evanston

Southwestern WY Alcohol
  Rehabilitation Association
1235 Uinta Street
Evanston, WY 82930
(307) 789-0734
Hotline: (307) 789-0737

Gillette

Wyoming Regional Counseling
  Center
900 West 6th Street
Gillette, WY 82716
(307) 687-5517
Hotline: (307) 686-9229

Rock Springs

Southwest Counseling Service
1124 College Road
Rock Springs, WY 82901
(307) 362-1848
Hotline: (307) 332-2231

Sheridan

Northern Wyoming Mental
  Health Center
1221 West 5th Street
Sheridan, WY 82801
(307) 674-4405

Don't wait for your ship to come in; swim out to it.
Anonymous

11

Suggested Reading

There are many books about the various aspects of alcoholism. This listing is by no means complete but will get you started.

Alcoholics Anonymous, *Living Sober*, A.A. World Services Inc., New York, 1975.

Bill W. and others, *Alcoholics Anonymous*, A.A. World Services Inc., New York, 1955.

Drews, Toby Rice, *Getting Them Sober: Volume One*, Bridge Publishing, Inc., South Plainfield, NJ, 1980.

Drews, Toby Rice, *Getting Them Sober: Volume Two*, Bridge Publishing, Inc., South Plainfield, NJ, 1983.

Johnson, Vernon, *Intervention: How To Help Someone Who Doesn't Want Help*, Johnson Institute Press, Minneapolis, 1986.

Milam, James R. and Ketcham, Katherine, *Under The Influence: A Guide To The Myths And Realities Of Alcoholism*, Madrona Publishers, Seattle, 1981.

Mueller, L. Ann, M.D. and Ketcham, Katherine, *Recovering: How To Get And Stay Sober*, Bantam, New York, 1987.

Robertson, Nan, *Getting Better: Inside Alcoholics Anonymous*, Ballantine Books, New York, 1988.

Rogers, Ronald L. and McMillin, Chandler Scott, *Freeing Someone You Love From Alcohol And Other Drugs*, Price Stern Sloan, Inc., Los Angeles, 1989.

Notes

Notes

Order Form

Here's how to get your own copy of *Alcohol Abuse: How To Help A Loved One:*

- Purchase a copy at your local bookstore

- Call 1-800-35-BOOKS (1-800-352-6657) 24 hours a day, 7 days a week. Visa and Mastercard accepted.

- Mail check or money order for $12.95 *(includes shipping & handling)* to:

Thunderbird Press
4130 N. Goldwater Boulevard
Suite 120
Scottsdale, AZ 85251

Please send_____copies of *Alcohol Abuse: How To Help A Loved One* to:

Name_____

Address_____

City_____State_____Zip_____

Enclosed is $12.95 per book.

Quantity discounts are available.
For details, please contact Publishers Distribution Service (PDS)
TEL: (616) 276-5196 or FAX: (616) 276-5197 for bulk orders.